Practice Test #1

Practice Questions

1. A patient with an acute depressive episode is brought into the ED by her family. What is your priority?
    a. Administering a new prescription for sertraline (*Zoloft*) and counseling her about its proper use
    b. Assessing her for suicidal ideation
    c. Admitting her to the psychiatric unit without her consent
    d. Referring her to a psychologist for counseling

2. Which of the following is not a symptom of an acute panic attack?
    a. Shortness of breath
    b. Intense fear/anxiety
    c. Diarrhea
    d. Vomiting

3. The police bring a young man into the ED for evaluation after becoming violent at a local shop. The patient is handcuffed to the bed, and he appears calm. His family, who has accompanied the young man to the ED, confides in you that he is schizophrenic. Which action is appropriate?
    a. Removing the handcuffs to escort him to the bathroom
    b. Administering haloperidol 5 mg IM
    c. Placing the patient in a private room
    d. Discharging the patient against medical advice when the patient demands to be released

4. An elderly woman is brought into the ED with a suspected overdose. Her family found her unconscious in her bathroom with an empty bottle of *Tylenol* nearby. They state that she has been depressed since losing her husband of 58 years, only 2 months ago. Which drug is appropriate for a *Tylenol* overdose?
    a. Naloxone
    b. Flumazenil
    c. Diazepam
    d. N-acetylcysteine

5. A 15-year-old adolescent girl is brought into the ED after fainting in school. After her initial workup, you begin to suspect that she is bulimic. What physical signs or laboratory results would you NOT expect to see in a patient with bulimia?
    a. Emaciated appearance
    b. Dental carries
    c. Knuckle scars
    d. Electrolyte imbalance

6. A 16-year-old adolescent girl is brought to the ED with severe right-sided abdominal and pelvic pain. She is also complaining of right shoulder pain. Last menstrual period was 6 weeks ago. What medication should you anticipate administering?
   a. Rho(D) immune globulin human (RhoGAM)
   b. Methotrexate
   c. Magnesium Sulfate
   d. Oxytocin

7. A 28-week-old infant is brought in to the ED after an unexpected home delivery. The baby's weight is 2 lb, and she is in cardiac arrest. The doctor orders 0.2 mL/kg of epinephrine to be administered IV. What is the dose of medication that you administer?
   a. 0. 88mL
   b. 8.8 mL
   c. 0.18 mL
   d. 1.8 mL

8. Which of the following is an inappropriate intervention for a woman in labor with a prolapsed cord?
   a. Placing the patient in the Trendelenburg position.
   b. Administering oxygen.
   c. Applying pressure to the presenting part to relieve pressure on the cord.
   d. Placing the patient on her right side.

9. Which of the following should be collected as part of a rape/sexual assault kit?
   a. Assault history
   b. Vaginal, mouth, and rectal samples
   c. Informed consent
   d. All of the above

10. A woman presents with vaginal itching and discharge, odor, and swelling. Testing with nitrazine paper indicates a pH of 4.8. Which medication should you recommend (as prescribed)?
   a. Hydrocortisone cream vaginally twice a day
   b. Clindamycin vaginal cream and Metronidazole
   c. Nonprescription antifungal creams
   d. Fluconazole tablet in 1 dose

11. Which of the following symptoms would not be present in a patient with kidney stones?
   a. Fever
   b. Diaphoresis
   c. Hematuria
   d. Flank, abdominal, or pelvic pain

12. Strategies to reduce the incidence of urinary tract infections in a patient with an indwelling urinary catheter do NOT include:
   a. Irrigating the bladder frequently
   b. Using a closed-drainage system
   c. Inserting and caring for a catheter using aseptic techniques
   d. Gently cleaning the urinary meatus each day

13. Which of the following is not a symptom of acute prostatitis?
    a. Fever
    b. Low back pain
    c. Incontinence
    d. Urinary frequency or painful urination

14. A 16-year-old adolescent boy comes into the ED after being found unconscious at home. An empty bottle of diazepam is found next to his bedside. Which of the following is not an appropriate treatment?
    a. Administration of flumazenil as ordered
    b. Frequent monitoring of respiratory and neurological status
    c. Administration of charcoal
    d. Administration of fomepizole as ordered

15. What is the drug of choice for *Salmonella* infection in a severely ill patient?
    a. Levofloxacin
    b. Metronidazole
    c. Penicillin G
    d. Erythromycin

16. What position should you place a patient about to undergo gastric lavage because of ingestion of a toxic substance?
    a. Trendelenburg
    b. Left lateral decubitus with head down
    c. Left lateral decubitus with head elevated
    d. Seated

17. A patient is brought into the ED with full thickness burns covering the front of his trunk, arms, and face. Which electrolyte levels should the nurse pay particularly close attention to? (There may be more than one response.)
    a. Phosphorus
    b. Glucose
    c. Sodium
    d. Potassium
    e. Chloride
    f. Calcium

18. A police officer finds an older man wandering the streets with disorientation and slurred speech. He is brought to the ED to be evaluated. Blood alcohol level is found to be 0.21%. The rest of his drug screen is negative. He is sleeping, but easily arousable. Vital signs remain normal. What is the appropriate intervention?
    a. Immediate gastric lavage
    b. Allow him to "sleep it off," but check on him frequently
    c. Discharge from the ED
    d. Endotracheal intubation

19. Which of the following should be avoided when treating a patient with hypothermia and frostbite?
   a. Debridement of hemorrhagic blisters
   b. Debridement of clear blisters
   c. Application of aloe vera cream
   d. Initially rewarming the affected area rapidly in a warm water bath until the frostbitten area is red and supple

20. Which of the following is not a symptom of Lyme disease?
   a. Flu-like symptoms
   b. Bull's eye rash
   c. Joint pain
   d. Diarrhea

21. A 2-year-old child is brought into the ED with lethargy, vomiting, and severe diarrhea. The parents report that the child swallowed a bottle of children's vitamins while out of sight of the parents. Which medication should you anticipate administering?
   a. Flumazenil
   b. Naloxone
   c. Deferoxamine
   d. N-acetylcysteine

22. A young man comes into the ED with a respiratory rate of 9 breaths per minute and a blood pressure of 82/49. He is disoriented, but awake and following commands. What is his score using the revised trauma scoring system?
   a. 9
   b. 10
   c. 11
   d. 12

23. What is the preferred site for a 2-year-old child requiring intraosseous infusion?
   a. The sternum
   b. Proximal tibia
   c. Pelvic bone
   d. Clavicle

24. A patient is brought into the ED with sudden onset of confusion, angioedema, and bronchospasm during lunch with a colleague. Patient is hypotensive. What medication should not be administered?
   a. Albuterol
   b. Methylprednisolone
   c. Atropine
   d. Diphenhydramine

25. Which of the following is not a sign that a patient is going into shock?
   a. Decreased urinary output
   b. Hypertension
   c. Hypotension
   d. Tachycardia

- 6 -

26. A patient in hypovolemic shock has lost approximately 1,750 mL of fluid. How is the shock classified?
    a. Class I
    b. Class II
    c. Class III
    d. Class IV

27. You are taking care of a patient that is in severe shock that has just arrived in the ED, after he was found unresponsive after a fall from a bridge. The patient has a decreased preload, decreased SVR, and an increased cardiac output. The patient has warm, dry skin and bradycardia. You suspect:
    a. Hypovolemic shock
    b. Neurogenic shock
    c. Cardiogenic Shock
    d. Anaphylaxis

28. Autotransfusion is contraindicated in which of the following clinical situations?
    a. The injury/wound occurred 2 hours ago.
    b. The patient has a cancerous tumor in the location where the blood to be transfused would be taken.
    c. The blood has not been heparinized.
    d. A commercial autotransfusion kit is not available.

29. Which of the following lab results would you expect to see in a patient who is in septic shock?
    a. Increased BUN
    b. Elevated platelets
    c. Decreased lactic acid
    d. Decrease in bilirubin

30. Which of the following should be administered if IV fluids are insufficient in correcting hypotension?
    a. Dobutamine
    b. Atropine
    c. Epinephrine
    d. Dopamine

31. Which of the following signs is a symptom of peritonitis?
    a. Psoas sign
    b. Blumberg sign
    c. Obturator sign
    d. Currant jelly stool

32. Your patient has been receiving IV clindamycin via home health for infection and has returned to the ED today with abdominal pain and diarrhea. She has now been diagnosed with *Clostridium difficile* infection. Which of the following would not apply to this patient?
    a. Education about her new medication, Metronidazole
    b. Education about continuing Clindamycin
    c. Education about contact precautions for her to share with her family
    d. Education about using vigorous soap and water for frequent hand sanitation

33. A patient presents with a chronic cough at night, earache, dysphagia, hoarseness, epigastric pain. What diagnosis would the nurse begin to suspect?
    a. Peptic ulcer
    b. Cholecystitis
    c. Pancreatitis
    d. Gastroesophageal reflux disease (GERD)

34. A 1-year-old child presents to the ED with episodes of what appear to be severe abdominal pain. His mother says that he has been lethargic and that his belly is bigger than normal. You observe the child pulling his knees to his chest during one such episode. Upon exam, you note a sausage-shaped mass in his abdomen. What do you suspect?
    a. Intussusception
    b. Appendicitis
    c. Hernia
    d. Acute constipation

35. A young woman is brought into the ED after a motor vehicle accident. She is complaining of severe pain in her abdomen and left shoulder. Upon exam, you note ecchymosis around her navel. You should be most concerned about:
    a. Intestinal perforation
    b. Pancreatic contusion
    c. Splenic rupture
    d. GI hemorrhage

36. When is FAST indicated?
    a. Suspected liver laceration
    b. Suspected cervical injury
    c. Rule out pregnancy
    d. Assess intracranial pressure

37. When inserting an ordered nasogastric tube, the tube insertion length is estimated to be:
    a. The distance from the earlobe to the xiphoid process + the distance from the earlobe to the nose tip + 5 cm
    b. The distance from the earlobe to the xiphoid process + the distance from the earlobe to the nose tip + 15 cm
    c. The distance from the earlobe to the xiphoid process + the distance from the earlobe to the nose tip + 25 cm
    d. The distance from the earlobe to the xiphoid process + the distance from the earlobe to the nose tip + 35 cm

38. A young child is brought into the ED with a fever. His parents report that he is restless, has been drooling, and that his voice "sounds funny." You observe the child sitting up and leaning slightly forward. His mouth is open and the tongue is protruding. He denies coughing. He is pale and slightly cyanotic. What is the likely diagnosis?
    a. Acute tracheitis
    b. Peritonsillar abscess
    c. Croup
    d. Acute epiglottitis

39. What is the primary medication give to a patient with temporal arteritis to prevent blindness?
    a. Mannitol 1 to 2 g/kg
    b. Prednisone 60 mg once daily
    c. Prednisone 60 mg once daily and acyclovir 400mg five times daily
    d. Phenytoin 100 mg three times daily

40. A patient presents with a hyphema, with blood occupying less than one-third of the eye chamber, caused by blunt trauma. Which of the following would not be an appropriate nursing intervention?
    a. Patch for injured eye
    b. NSAIDS for pain
    c. Topical steroids
    d. anti-glaucoma topical meds, if increased IOP.

41. Which of the following actions is inappropriate for handling an avulsed tooth prior to reimplantation?
    a. Transportation of the tooth from the scene of the accident in a cup of milk.
    b. Clean the tooth thoroughly with Hanks solution.
    c. Irrigate the socket with normal saline.
    d. Gently trim the nerve fibers hanging from the bottom of the tooth to facilitate new growth.

42. You are evaluating a patient with suspected retinal detachment, which of the following do you not expect to find on history and assessment?
    a. Eye pain
    b. Loss of central vision
    c. Seeing floaters
    d. Photopsia

43. What is the correct term for a study that demonstrates a confirmed cause-and-effect relationship?
    a. External validity
    b. Internal validity
    c. Sample size
    d. Sample selection

44. Which is not an appropriate strategy for managing stress associated with a critical incident?
    a. A focus on educating the staff about peer coping and support strategies
    b. A group debriefing 12 to 48 hours after the incident
    c. Making mental health counseling available for everyone involved
    d. Brief meeting during the incident to discuss posttraumatic stress disorder

45. Which of the following tasks would be appropriately delegated to an unlicensed patient care technician?
    a. Assisting a stable patient to ambulate to the restroom.
    b. Changing wound dressings on a sacral decubitus while bathing a stable patient.
    c. Checking on a patient after her first dose of morphine for pain.
    d. Transporting an unstable patient to a scheduled CT scan

46. A young woman comes into the ED and is given a new diagnosis of HIV. The young woman begs the nurse not to tell anyone. How should the nurse handle her reporting responsibilities?
    a. Report the diagnosis to both the CDC and the state, but only on the condition that you do not provide her name
    b. Respect her wishes and not report the diagnosis on the basis of patient confidentiality
    c. File the report according to state and federal guidelines
    d. Speak with your nurse manager for guidance

47. An elderly patient on a ventilator is brought into the ED. His children wish that he be removed from life support. The patient does not have any legal documents dictating his wishes or assigning a health care proxy. What should the nurse do?
    a. Respect the family's request and arrange with the doctor to remove life support
    b. Nothing; the patient did not express his wishes to be removed from mechanical ventilation
    c. Wait a few days and see if the patient improves
    d. Speak with the nurse manager about bringing the case to the ethics committee, or about the institution's policies pertaining to the situation

48. A 21-year-old woman is brought into the ED with suspected facial fractures. She is accompanied by her boyfriend. Upon exam, you note several bruises in various stages of healing on the woman's wrists and arms. Which action should be performed first?
    a. Calling the police
    b. Isolating the patient from her boyfriend and asking her if she is being abused
    c. Providing information about domestic abuse
    d. Treating her fractures and discharging her home

49. You are caring for a patient post motor vehicle accident, with a cleared C-Spine, pain rating 8/10, and with an ICP of 21. Which of the following is an inappropriate intervention?
    a. Medications to manage pain as necessary
    b. Administration of a diuretic such as mannitol or furosemide
    c. Mechanical ventilation as necessary
    d. Positioning the patient flat on her back

50. A patient comes in to the ED after a motor vehicle accident. During the neurological assessment, you note that his eyes open to painful stimuli, he is not verbal, and he moves in a withdrawal motion in response to pain. What is his Glasgow Coma Scale (GCS)?
    a. 5
    b. 6
    c. 7
    d. 8

51. You are caring for a patient with suspected increased ICP following blunt trauma to the head that just arrived in the ER. Her GCS when the paramedics found her was 12 and is still 12. Currently in sinur rhythm, blood pressure 150/62. Which of the following is an appropriate intervention to decrease ICP?
   a. Nasotracheal intubation if ventilation required.
   b. Keep the head of the bed flat to promote drainage.
   c. Begin hyperventilation of the patient now.
   d. Analgesia as needed.

52. A patient comes into the ED with a severe headache and stiffness in the back of her neck, facial paralysis, and visual changes. A CT scan confirms that the patient has a subarachnoid hemorrhage. Which of the following would not be indicated for treatment?
   a. Giving ordered antihypertensives
   b. Preparing the patient for immediate intubation
   c. Observing for signs of re-bleeding
   d. Giving ant-seizure medications as ordered.

53. A patient with generalized seizure disorder was brought to the ER by ambulance with her college dorm mate. The patient is now confused, disoriented, and experiencing nausea and vomiting. What education is appropriate at this time?
   a. Explain that this behavior is a normal part of the tonic period.
   b. Explain that this behavior is a normal part of the clonic period
   c. Explain that this behavior is normal following a seizure.
   d. Explain that this is abnormal behavior and you need the dorm mate to help you get in contact with the patient's parents.

54. What portion of the spinal cord is likely to be damaged in a patient with loss of bowel or bladder control and loss of sensation and motor ability in the lower extremities?
   a. Cauda equina
   b. Central cord
   c. Anterior cord
   d. Posterior cord

55. Corticosteroids should be started how soon after a spinal cord injury?
   a. Within 24 hours
   b. Within 12 hours
   c. Within 8 hours
   d. Within 1 hour

56. An elderly patient is brought into the ED with worsening dementia after his diagnosis of Alzheimer disease several months ago. You are counseling the patient's daughter and caretaker about his new prescription, memantine (*Namenda*). Which nonprescription medication should be avoided in someone taking memantine?
   a. Acetaminophen
   b. Nonprescription cough syrups
   c. Ibuprofen
   d. Antacids containing calcium

57. A 25-year-old woman presents to the ED with worsening balance and coordination, speech difficulties, and loss of central vision. She has had the symptoms on and off for several weeks but fell this afternoon, which is what brought her in for evaluation. What do you suspect?

a. Multiple sclerosis
b. Stroke
c. Amyotrophic lateral sclerosis (ALS)
d. Myasthenia gravis

58. Tissue plasminogen activator (tPA) is contraindicated in which patient?

a. A 79-year-old man with a platelet count of 250,000/cu mm
b. An 87-year-old woman who had a stroke 2 hours ago
c. A 65-year-old man with mild and controlled hypertension
d. A 92-year-old man who had a stroke 2 weeks ago

59. The nurse places her hands on the back of the patient's head and slightly flexes the patient's head forward. If the patient has pain or increased resistance during this maneuver it is a symptom of all of the following except:

a. bacterial meningitis
b. subarachnoid hemorrhage
c. leukemia
d. epidural hematoma

60. A 45 year old woman is diagnosed with an ischemic brain attack. She has been intubated due to neurologic status and respiratory distress. She has a history of hypertension (currently controlled with medication), seizures (controlled with medication and without an active seizure in more than 5 years), and is on medication for a peptic ulcer. Her daughter, an LVN, asks if she will receive the fibrinolytics that the doctor ordered. Your answer is that we can talk more about this to the physician but in most cases:

a. No, she can't because hypertension is an absolute contraindication.
b. No, she can't because seizures are an absolute contraindication.
c. No, she can't because peptic ulcers are an absolute contraindication.
d. Yes, she can, while she has some relative contraindications, she doesn't have any absolute contraindications.

61. You are assessing a patient for abdominal pain after a motor vehicle accident. You ask for her pain score (between 0 [no pain] and 10 [excruciating pain]) and she says "8." However, the patient is sitting up in bed and not displaying any physical signs of discomfort. How do you document her pain score?

a. 2
b. 4
c. 6
d. 8

62. A woman in labor is brought into the ED by ambulance after going into labor in her car. She is demanding to be brought to a different hospital where her obstetrician has privileges. Upon exam, she is found to be 8 cm dilated. How should the transfer be handled?
    a. Transfer the patient to the other hospital, according to her wishes
    b. Transfer the patient up to the obstetrics unit upstairs to deliver her baby
    c. Deliver the baby in the ED and then transfer the patient upstairs to recover
    d. Transfer the woman and her baby (born without complications) to the other hospital after delivery

63. After a major mass casualty incident, patients are being brought into the ED to be triaged. How would you assign a young woman with a dislocated right shoulder, amputated right thumb, and no other apparent injuries?
    a. Red
    b. Yellow
    c. Green
    d. Black

64. You receive a medication from the pharmacy that does not match what the physician prescribed for the patient. What should you do?
    a. Check the order again and then speak with the ordering physician to confirm what he prescribed and then notify the pharmacy if a mistake was made.
    b. Notify the pharmacy of the mistake immediately
    c. Administer the medication that was delivered; you must have misheard the physician when he was giving you the order
    d. Double-check the written order against the delivered medication and then speak with a pharmacist about the mistake.

65. An elderly woman is brought into the ED after she was found wandering in the street, confused. You are concerned that she may get out of bed and walk away from the unit. What should you do?
    a. Apply a vest restraint to keep her in bed
    b. Administer haloperidol 4 mg IV as ordered
    c. Check on the patient as frequently as possible
    d. Assign one of the unlicensed personnel or volunteers to sit with her

66. A 20-year-old woman is brought is into the ED after a seizure. The physician orders a single dose of phenytoin 10 mg/kg via slow IV infusion, at a rate of 45 mg/min. Her admission weight was 120 lb. How long should the infusion take?
    a. 12 minutes
    b. 27 minutes
    c. 59 minutes
    d. 82 minutes

67. Which of the following is included in the 5 basic rights of medication administration? (More than one answer may apply.)
    a. Right patient
    b. Right order of medications
    c. Right dose of medication
    d. All of the above

68. What type of personal protective equipment (PPE) is necessary when changing the dressing on a stage IV sacral pressure ulcer?
    a. Gloves
    b. Gown and gloves
    c. Gloves and mask
    d. Gown, mask, and gloves

69. To extend viability, an amputated limb should be cooled to what temperature before reattachment?
    a. 0°C
    b. 4°C
    c. 14°C
    d. 20°C

70. What is the best way to remove a bee stinger?
    a. Soak the part in warm water and gently slide the stinger out of the skin
    b. Grasp the stinger firmly and pull from the skin
    c. Gently scrape a sharp instrument over the area to scrape the stinger out of the skin
    d. Apply ice to the area and, when numb, remove the stinger using tweezers

71. What should the nurse do with a tick once it has been removed from a patient who has been bitten?
    a. Wash it down the sink
    b. Place in a medical waste bag and dispose with the medical waste
    c. Place the tick in a plastic bag in the freezer
    d. Kill it and place in the garbage

72. All of the following are symptoms of compartment syndrome except:
    a. Numbness and tingling of the affected area
    b. Swelling
    c. Decreased pulses
    d. Pain relieved by Tylenol

73. A positive Tinel test indicates what condition?
    a. Carpal tunnel syndrome
    b. Compartment syndrome
    c. Costochondritis
    d. Bursitis

74. Which of the following is not a recommended treatment for a shoulder dislocation?
    a. Reduction
    b. Immobilization
    c. Use of heating pad for pain relief
    d. Use of a cold compress to reduce swelling

75. Which bacteria is the most common cause of infectious arthritis?
    a. Rubella
    b. Chlamydia
    c. Neisseria gonorrhoeae
    d. Clostridium

76. A patient presents with sudden swelling, edema and pain in a joint. What level of uric acid (in addition to results from the clinical exam) would help confirm a diagnosis of gout?
   a. Below 7 mg/dL
   b. Above 7 mg/dL
   c. Below 70 mg/dL
   d. Above 70 mg/dL

77. When should heat be applied to a strained muscle?
   a. Immediately after the injury
   b. In the first 48 hours after the injury
   c. After the first 48 hours since the injury has passed
   d. Never

78. When assessing venous refill time on a patient, what time is considered to be indicative of a venous occlusion?
   a. Greater than 2 to 3 seconds
   b. Greater than 5 seconds
   c. Greater than 10 seconds
   d. Greater than 20 seconds

79. On a scale from 0 to 4, how should normal pulse intensity be documented?
   a. 1
   b. 2
   c. 3
   d. 4

80. A private room with monitored negative pressure is appropriate for the patient with which infection?
   a. Measles
   b. Pertussis
   c. Influenza
   d. Pneumonia

81. What lab values would you expect to see in a patient who is in disseminated intravascular coagulation (DIC)?
   a. Increased fibrinogen, prolonged PT/PTT, increased platelets
   b. Decreased fibrinogen, prolonged PT/PTT, increased platelets
   c. Decreased fibrinogen, prolonged PT/PTT, decreased platelets
   d. Increased fibrinogen, prolonged PT/PTT, decreased platelets

82. A young child is brought into the ED with epistaxis and bruising. He has type A hemophilia. Which of the following is the priority nursing intervention at this time?
   a. Provide emotional support for the patient and his family.
   b. Give analgesics as needed.
   c. Give Factor VII.
   d. Apply pressure by pinching the nose and having the child lean forward.

- 15 -

83. A patient with AIDS has presented to the ER with fever, a dry cough, dyspnea and chills. Chest x-ray shows diffuse opacities. The nurse and physician have completed their assessments. What is the priority nursing intervention?
    a. Checking CD4 count.
    b. Giving TMP-SMX IV as ordered.
    c. Giving antiretroviral medications.
    d. Collect blood and sputum cultures.

84. Which of the following is not a lab value that you would see in a patient with hyperglycemic hyperosmolar nonketotic syndrome (HHNK)?
    a. Blood glucose above 600 mg/dL
    b. Increased BUN
    c. Increased creatinine
    d. Decreased serum osmolality

85. A patient comes into the ED with enlarged, painless lymph nodes, fever, and weakness. A blood smear shows the presence of Reed-Sternberg cells. What condition does this patient likely have?
    a. Leukocytosis
    b. Hodgkin lymphoma
    c. Non-Hodgkin lymphoma
    d. Leukemia

86. What are the normal white blood cell counts for a neonate?
    a. 9,000 to 30,000/mm3
    b. 5,000 to 15,000/mm3
    c. 6,000 to 18, 000/mm3
    d. 2,000 to 10,000/mm3

87. Which of the following is not recommended treatment for a patient infected with scabies?
    a. Permethrin cream to entire body
    b. Antihistamines
    c. Frequent betadine baths
    d. Doxycycline

88. A patient with a painless chancre on his genitals has which phase of syphilis?
    a. Primary
    b. Secondary
    c. Tertiary
    d. Latent

89. A nurse caring for a patient in the ED with Chlamydia knows that she should educate the patient about all of the following regarding this STD *except*:
    a. Doxycycline is an antibiotic of choice for treatment
    b. Many patients with Chlamydia are coinfected with gonorrhea
    c. A patient with chlamydia must avoid sexual contact for 3 months
    d. Treating the infected person's partner is crucial to avoid reinfection

90. A patient has been brought into the ER by ambulance in cardiac arrest. Medications that were able to be given through ETT have been given, but the physician is unable despite multiple attempts to secure a central venous line to give further medications. The physician gives order to use the AV fistula to give emergency medications. What is the proper solution for prepping the skin before accessing an arteriovenous (AV) fistula?
   a. Alcohol prep
   b. Do not follow this order, you may not access an AV fistula for any reason but dialysis.
   c. Betadine
   d. Povidone-iodine

91. What is the age range in which febrile seizures are most common?
   a. Birth through 6 months
   b. 6 months through 5 years
   c. 5 years through 10 years
   d. 70 years and older

92. Phenobarbital 15 mg/kg IV is ordered for a young child weighing 16 lb who is having febrile seizures. What dose should the child receive?
   a. 109 mg
   b. 240 mg
   c. 528 mg
   d. 1,056 mg

93. What is the proper depth to which an endotracheal tube should be inserted when intubating a 4-year-old girl?
   a. 12 cm
   b. 14 cm
   c. 16 cm
   d. 21 cm

94. Which of the following group of lab values indicate respiratory failure?
   a. PaCO2 70 mm Hg, PaO2 50 mm Hg
   b. PaCO2 50 mm Hg, PaO2 85 mm Hg
   c. PaCO2 40 mm Hg, PaO2 80 mm Hg
   d. PaCO2 40 mm Hg, PaO2 85 mm Hg

95. What should be the first step in medical treatment of a young child in status asthmaticus?
   a. Immediate intubation
   b. Administration of albuterol
   c. Administration of theophylline
   d. Administer the child's emergency inhaler and monitor for its effectiveness

96. Which bacterium is most commonly implicated in children with tracheitis?
   a. Clostridium
   b. Influenza
   c. Haemophilus influenzae
   d. Staphylococcus *aureus*

97. Which of the following is NOT indicative of respiratory alkalosis?
  a. Low PaCO2
  b. Normal sodium bicarbonate
  c. Decreased pH
  d. Increased pH

98. What structures of the lungs are affected with interstitial pneumonia?
  a. The bronchi
  b. The bronchioles
  c. The alveoli
  d. The lower lobes

99. A patient presents to the ED with decreased breath sounds, hemodynamic instability, and tracheal deviation. What does the nurse suspect?
  a. Spontaneous Pneumothorax
  b. Cardiac Tamponade
  c. Traumatic
  d. Tension

100. Having which of the following conditions puts a patient at greater risk for respiratory acidosis?
  a. Guillain-Barré
  b. Croup
  c. Bronchitis
  d. Hypothyroidism

101. When a clinician is applying pressure to the cricoid using the thumb and fore finger during a rapid sequence intubation, which of the following has not likely been done yet?
  a. Sellick manuver
  b. Administration of paralytics
  c. Administration of sedatives
  d. Capnography

102. Which type of ventilation is most appropriate for a patient with congestive heart failure?
  a. Bilevel positive airway pressure (BiPAP)
  b. Continuous positive airway pressure (CPAP)
  c. Tracheostomy
  d. Laryngeal mask airway (LMA)

103. The nurse giving you report at shift change tells you that the patient's blood gas results were normal. When you are looking at the results, which correlate with this report regarding the PaO_2 value?
  a. 55 mm Hg
  b. 65 mm Hg
  c. 75 mm Hg
  d. 85 mm Hg

104. A patient with a new prescription for ipratropium should be counseled to notify his physician if he notices:
    a. Vision changes
    b. Nausea
    c. Dry mouth or nose
    d. Nosebleeds

105. A 16-year-old adolescent girl comes into the ED with shortness of breath, chest pain, and rapid heart rate. She discloses that she is an occasional smoker and was recently given a prescription for birth control pills, which her parents do not know she is taking. What do you begin to suspect?
    a. Pneumothorax
    b. Pulmonary embolism
    c. Congestive heart failure
    d. Pleural effusion

106. You just receive the results of an ordered arterial blood gas: pH 7.2, $PaCO_2$ 50 mm Hg, H_2CO_3 26 mEq/L. You suspect:
    a. Respiratory acidosis
    b. Respiratory alkalosis
    c. Metabolic acidosis
    d. Metabolic alkalosis

107. If a patient came into the ED after a motor vehicle accident and an x-ray confirms two broken ribs on the left, which of the following should you be more alert for when monitoring the patient:
    a. Liver laceration
    b. Small bowel laceration
    c. Splenic rupture
    d. Rupture of the appendix

108. Where is the V4 lead placed when administering a 12-lead ECG?
    a. The 4th intercostal space on the right sternal border
    b. The 4th intercostal space on the left sternal border
    c. The 5th intercostal space, midclavicular on the right
    d. The 5th intercostal space, midclavicular on the left

109. Where would a right sided V6 lead be placed when administering an ECG?
    a. The 4th intercostal space on the right sternal border
    b. The 5th intercostal space, midclavicular on the right
    c. The 5th intercostal space at the right midaxillary line
    d. The 5th intercostal space at the right anterior axillary line

110. Determine the significance of the mean arterial pressure (MAP) for a patient with a blood pressure of 100/64.
    a. This is a measure of cardiac output and peripheral resistance, and this is a normal value.
    b. This is a measure of cardiac output and peripheral resistance, and this an abnormal value.
    c. This is a measure of heart rate and stroke volume, and this is a normal value.
    d. This is a measure of heart rate and stroke volume, and this is an abnormal value.

111. An unstable patient is about to have an arterial line placed. The Allen's test is performed. The patient has a positive result in the left hand and a negative result in the right hand. Where should the arterial line be placed?
    a. Left radial
    b. Right Radial
    c. Femoral
    d. It is not appropriate to place an arterial line in this patient.

112. When using length-based resuscitation tape, where should the red end of the tape be placed?
    a. In line with the top of the child's head
    b. In line with the axilla
    c. In line with the child's nipples
    d. In line with the umbilicus

113. What position should a patient who is about to undergo pericardiocentesis be positioned?
    a. Supine
    b. On her right side
    c. Chest elevated 45 degrees
    d. Trendelenburg

114. What type of aneurysm occurs when 3 layers of the aortic wall are bulging?
    a. True aortic aneurysm
    b. Dissecting aneurysm
    c. Fusiform aneurysm
    d. False aneurysm

115. According to the American Heart Association (AHA), what is the ideal total volume of medication (mixed with diluent, if necessary) to be administered via the endotracheal route to an adult?
    a. 1 mL
    b. 2 mL
    c. 5 mL
    d. 10 mL

116. You are caring for a patient in Class III heart failure, with atrial fibrillation, and diabetes. The patient had a new medication started yesterday by her primary care doctor but she is unable to tell you which one, by looking at her home medication list. She tells you her list is a combination of medications that are managed by her primary care doctor, cardiologist, and endocrinologist. You review the patient's medication list and see Lisinopril, Digoxin, Furosemide, Coumadin, Captopril, Metformin and Insulin. What is wrong with the patient's medication list?
    a. Digoxin should not be used with an ACE inhibitor.
    b. There is nothing wrong, and this is an appropriate medication list.
    c. There are two diabetic medications, and this should be investigated further.
    d. There are two ACE inhibitors, and this should be investigated further.

117. Which of the following medications would be appropriately used to convert a patient in atrial flutter to a sinus rhythm?
    a. Digoxin
    b. Quinidine
    c. Lidocaine
    d. Adenosine

118. When would you expect myoglobin levels to begin to rise after a patient has had an myocardial infarction (MI)?
    a. Immediately
    b. Within 1 to 3 hours
    c. Within 12 hours
    d. Within 24 hours

119. How should you position a patient's head when assessing jugular venous pressure?
    a. Elevated 45 degrees and turned to the right
    b. Elevated 45 degrees and turned to the left
    c. In line with the patient's body and turned to the right
    d. In line with the patient's body and turned to the left

120. Where is the initial incision made during an emergency thoracotomy?
    a. Anterolaterally in the 2nd left intercostal space
    b. Anterolaterally in the 3rd left intercostal space
    c. Anterolaterally in the 4th left intercostal space
    d. Anterolaterally in the 5th left intercostal space

121. Which of the following adverse effects should you counsel a patient with a new prescription for simvastatin to report immediately to his physician?
    a. Nausea/vomiting
    b. Stomach discomfort
    c. Frequent heartburn
    d. Yellowing of the skin or eyes

122. What should you tell a patient with stable angina to do when they are having an episode?
a. Lie down and relax
b. Take an aspirin
c. Proceed to the ED immediately
d. Nothing; it will pass

123. You observe an ECG strip with the following attributes: regular rate of 42 bpm, regular P wave and QRS complex, PR interval of 0.15 seconds, and P to QRS ratio of 1:1. How would you label the rhythm?
a. Normal sinus rhythm
b. Sinus bradycardia
c. Sinus arrhythmia
d. First-degree AV block

124. You are caring for a patient with continuous cardiac monitoring after he came into the ED with chest pain and difficulty breathing. He has the following characteristics on his ECG: saw-toothed P waves, normal QRS shape, and a P to QRS ratio of 4:1. What do you suspect?
a. Atrial flutter
b. Atrial fibrillation
c. Ventricular dysrhythmia
d. Premature junctional contractions

125. Which of the following should a patient who is taking digoxin avoid?
a. Any and all types of alcohol
b. Caffeine
c. Prolonged periods of standing
d. Becoming dehydrated

126. A four-year-old boy is brought to the ED for sudden onset of fever, sore throat, and inspiratory stridor. As you assess the child, you note his agitated appearance, temperature of 104°F, and respiratory rate of 50/min. He appears anxious and is seated in a tripod position. The child has also been drooling for the past two hours and is unable to eat or drink. Of the following choices, the most important priority for the nurse caring for this child would be to
a. Immediately administer acetaminophen.
b. Anticipate orders for a strep test and swab the child's throat.
c. Prepare to administer racemic epinephrine.
d. Prepare to assist with intubation.

127. A man with a history of chronic hypertension and cigarette smoking is being evaluated in the ED for severe back pain and a pulsating sensation in the abdomen. An abdominal bruit is also present. Which one of the following is the most likely diagnosis?
a. myocardial infarction
b. pancreatitis
c. abdominal aortic aneurysm
d. gastritis

128. A 20-year-old woman arrives in the ED with a history of anorexia, intermittent crampy periumbilical pain, and recurrent diarrhea for the past several months. On a few occasions, she has also had fever along with the other symptoms. Sometimes she passes blood in her stools. A previous visit to her physician revealed negative stool cultures. She is now experiencing an acute flare-up. Further history reveals she has had episodes of joint pain and has lost 10 pounds in the past three weeks. On physical exam, the ED physician detects a perianal fistula. The joints are not swollen or tender, and the patient is currently afebrile. The patient's physical findings and symptoms are most consistent with a diagnosis of
    a. antibiotic-associated colitis
    b. diverticulitis
    c. Crohn's disease
    d. irritable bowel syndrome

129. An adult male comes into the ED appearing anxious and exhibiting unusual involuntary posturing. His eyes are gazing upward, and his neck is hyperextended and deviated to the left side. He recently started taking metoclopramide for gastroesophageal reflux disease (GERD), but he denies any other drug use. The ED physician has written orders for you to give the patient diphenhydramine 50 mg IV. Within 15 minutes of treatment, the symptoms fully resolve. You ask the physician what caused these symptoms, and she says it was a
    a. partial seizure
    b. dystonic reaction
    c. catatonic reaction
    d. transient ischemic attack

130. You are caring for a patient who sustained a lacerated frenulum of the upper lip as a result of a fall. Only the frenulum is involved. The injured area is slowly oozing blood. No other injuries are present. The most logical next step would be to
    a. reassure the patient that the injury is not serious.
    b. have absorbable suture material ready for repair.
    c. apply EMLA cream to the wound prior to discharge in order to ease the pain.
    d. prepare for cauterization of the wound.

131. Which one of the following statements is true about pulsus paradoxus?
    a. All patients with cardiac tamponade, by definition have pulsus paradoxus.
    b. When the pulsus paradoxus measurement is taken, the blood pressure cuff is deflated more slowly than when obtaining a routine blood pressure.
    c. Pulsus paradoxus measures an abnormally large decrease in systolic pressure on expiration.
    d. A patient is usually referred to a cardiologist to obtain a pulsus paradoxus measurement.

132. A 50-year-old woman arrives in the ED with right-upper-quadrant pain, nausea, vomiting, and a temperature of 100.8°F. The physician documents a positive Murphy's sign on her chart. Which one of the following is the most likely diagnosis?
    a. pancreatitis
    b. appendicitis
    c. cholecystitis
    d. gastroenteritis

133. A nurse in the ED is working with a physician who is examining a six-month-old baby with a cough. The physician orders a specimen for pertussis culture. The correct method for collection is to
   a. swab the pharynx with a rayon-tipped swab.
   b. draw 2 ml of blood and place it in a blood culture bottle.
   c. bulb suction mucus from a nostril and place it in a sterile container.
   d. swab the nasopharynx with a calcium alginate swab.

134. Which of the following is the best way to remove a tick?
   a. Grasp the tick with fine-tipped tweezers, twist two to three times, and then pull up on it.
   b. Grasp the tick with fine-tipped tweezers as close to the skin as possible, and pull straight up with steady pressure.
   c. Smother the tick with petroleum jelly, and then remove it manually after 10 minutes.
   d. Burn the tick off with a silver nitrate stick.

135. A patient has a potassium level of 7.8. Which one of the following electrocardiogram (ECG) changes would you expect to see?
   a. high-voltage P waves
   b. short QT interval
   c. sinus bradycardia
   d. peaked T waves

136. A 60-year-old woman has had surgery to remove a thyroid nodule. She now vocally complains of tingling and cramping in her hands and painful spasms in her right calf. The patient is anxious and irritable. Her blood pressure is 132/78, and her temperature is 98.8°F. Her ECG shows a normal sinus rhythm with a heart rate of 78 beats per minute and a prolongation of the QT interval. The most likely cause of these findings is
   a. hypocalcemia
   b. recurrent laryngeal nerve damage
   c. acute myocardial infarction (MI)
   d. long QT syndrome

137. A 65-year-old man sustained a severe direct blow to the occipital area in a car accident. Upon arrival in the ED, he is still unconscious. What part of the brain is most likely to show a contrecoup injury on imaging studies?
   a. occipital area
   b. cerebellum
   c. frontal lobe
   d. hippocampus

138. A pregnant woman at 38 weeks of gestation arrives in the ED in labor. On pelvic examination, the umbilical cord can be seen overlying the presenting part. The fetal heart monitor shows decelerations. All of the following are appropriate interventions EXCEPT
   a. Infuse 350 to 500 milliliters of warm normal saline into the bladder via a catheter.
   b. Place the patient in the knee–chest position.
   c. Push the cord out of the way with your hand and instruct the woman to push with the next contraction.
   d. Place the patient in the Trendelenburg position.

139. A patient has a thin, grayish-white vaginal discharge with mild itching. Which of the following vaginal problems is associated with a positive "whiff" test?
    a. bacterial vaginosis
    b. Candida albicans
    c. trichomonas
    d. atrophic vaginitis

140. A three-year-old child with no other history of recent illnesses arrives in the ED with a seven-day history of a purulent, blood-tinged, foul-smelling discharge from the right nostril. He has also been sneezing on occasion. The left nostril is clear. The child is not coughing or febrile. He seems mildly agitated because he can only breathe through one nostril. The most likely reason for these findings is
    a. foreign body in the right nostril
    b. sinus infection
    c. uncontrolled allergic rhinitis
    d. viral upper respiratory tract infection (URTI)

141. Which one of the following drugs is NOT commonly used in cardiopulmonary resuscitation?
    a. amiodarone
    b. verapamil
    c. lidocaine
    d. budesonide

142. Which one of the following fractures is most likely associated with physical abuse of a child who is not yet old enough to ambulate on his own?
    a. spiral leg fracture
    b. compressed vertebral fracture
    c. Monteggia fracture
    d. Galeazzi fracture

143. A nurse in the ED is assisting a physician with a 34-year-old man with an anterior nosebleed. In order to most effectively stop the nosebleed, the nurse should
    a. Prepare to assist the physician with nasal packing.
    b. Instruct the patient to tilt his head back.
    c. Pinch the nostrils together for at least 10 minutes.
    d. Apply an ice pack over the bridge of the nose.

144. A physician has ordered a 12-lead ECG on a 54-year-old patient. Which one of the following represents the correct positioning for precordial leads V4 and V5?
    a. V4 at the left midclavicular line in the fifth intercostal space; V5 horizontal to V4 at the left anterior axillary line
    b. V4 at the left anterior axillary line; V5 at the right sterna border in the fourth intercostal space
    c. V4 midway between V1 and V2; V5 horizontal to V6 at the left midaxillary line
    d. V4 anywhere along the right fifth intercostal space; V5 midway between V4 and V6

145. A patient with type 2 diabetes comes to the ED for evaluation of fatigue and muscle pain. He has been taking metformin for the past two years. He also admits to heavy alcohol consumption for the past week because of "personal problems." Which of the following would you be the most concerned about?
   a. hyperglycemia
   b. lactic acidosis
   c. cardiac dysrhythmia
   d. stress reaction

146. An undesired effect of a beta blocker given for treatment of heart failure in a patient with hypertension is:
   a. A decrease in blood pressure
   b. Pulsus alternans
   c. An increase in afterload
   d. Impotence

147. A 38-year-old woman received an IV dose of morphine in the ED. She is now experiencing respiratory suppression, constricted pupils, and she is unresponsive. Her pulses are easily detectable, and the respiratory rate is six per minute. You have already started administering oxygen. After securing the airway, which one of the following would be the most appropriate course of action?
   a. Call a code.
   b. Prepare to administer naloxone.
   c. Prepare to transfer her to the ICU.
   d. Insert a nasal airway.

148. Of the following, the most effective way to relieve asthma symptoms acutely is
   a. IV diphenhydramine
   b. three puffs orally of a fluticasone inhaler
   c. nebulized beta-2-receptor agonist
   d. leukotriene inhibitor

149. A patient arrives in the ED for vomiting, diarrhea, blurred vision, and paresthesias six hours after eating fish. The most likely cause of these symptoms is
   a. preformed *Staphylococcus aureus* toxin
   b. *Clostridium perfringens*
   c. ciguatoxin
   d. botulism

150. The classic appearance of a large pericardial effusion on x ray is
   a. a normal cardiac silhouette
   b. a boot-shaped silhouette
   c. tracheal deviation
   d. a "water bottle"-shaped cardiac silhouette

151. You are caring for a patient that arrested and is waiting to transfer to the cardiac ICU after resuscitation. A PA catheter was floated by the physician. The stroke volume is 50 ml/beat and the heart rate is 61 beats per minute. What do you know about the cardiac output?
    a. The cardiac output is normal.
    b. The cardiac output is high.
    c. The cardiac output is low.
    d. You can not calculate cardiac output with the given information.

152. The ED physician has ordered Narcan for an adult patient. Which one of the following is true about Narcan?
    a. The usual dose is 4 mg IV.
    b. The patient usually needs just one dose.
    c. It is a long-acting drug.
    d. The dose may need to be repeated.

153. What size of uncuffed endotracheal (ET) tube is most appropriate for an average four-year-old child?
    a. 3.0
    b. 4.0
    c. 5.0
    d. 6.0

154. A heparin overdose is treated with
    a. aminocaproic acid
    b. streptokinase
    c. protamine
    d. vitamin K

155. Which one of the following cerebrospinal (CSF) findings is consistent with Guillain-Barré syndrome?
    a. increased protein
    b. decreased protein
    c. increased glucose
    d. bacteria on Gram stain

156. A 48-year-old patient has tarry stools that tested positive for occult blood. This finding most often indicates bleeding from the
    a. descending colon
    b. upper-GI area
    c. rectum
    d. hemorrhoids

157. A patient with severe facial trauma has clear liquid draining from both nostrils. This is likely due to
    a. vasomotor rhinitis
    b. a cribriform plate fracture
    c. increased intracranial pressure
    d. respiratory arrest

158. Which one of the following are areas you may auscultate when assessing heart sounds (More than one answer may apply.)?
   a. aortic area
   b. purkinje area
   c. pulmonic area
   d. tricuspid area

159. The Broselow tape (More than one answer may apply.):
   a. Is used to determine resuscitation drug dosages in infants and small children.
   b. Provides sizes of resuscitation equipment.
   c. Is color coded.
   d. Measures the length of a child by starting at the head and stopping with the red-colored end at the heel.

160. The most common cause of hypoglycemia is
   a. adrenal insufficiency
   b. inborn errors of metabolism
   c. insulin reaction in diabetic patients
   d. excessive alcohol ingestion

161. You are assisting a physician in the placement of a femoral vein line in the ED. Which of these choices is true about femoral lines?
   a. They should always be considered contaminated.
   b. They are less likely to become infected than a subclavian line.
   c. They are not a good choice for venous access in a cardiac arrest.
   d. They are a good choice for long-term venous access.

162. A full-term six-week-old infant is brought to the ED by worried parents. They complain that the baby "seems nervous" because he startles too easily with sudden loud noises or if touched unexpectedly. The baby is otherwise healthy and had an uncomplicated delivery. You witness one of these episodes while talking with the parents. The baby threw out his arms, flexed the legs, and then adducted the arms into an embracing posture and let out a brief cry. In counseling the parents, you tell them
   a. These are infantile spasms.
   b. This is due to a chemical imbalance in the brain.
   c. This is a normal Moro reflex.
   d. The baby has cerebral palsy.

163. A patient presents to the ER with a pulmonary embolism. The patient is hemodynamically stable and the patient is not a candidate for thrombolytics due to history. The patient is started on anticoagulation therapy. Which one of the following is not true regarding anticoagulation therapy?
   a. Anticoagulation therapy can lyse existing clots.
   b. The goal of anticoagulation therapy is to achieve an INR of 2 to 2.5 .
   c. Anticoagulants are more likely than other medications to cause harm.
   d. Anticoagulants prevent clot propagation.

164. "Currant jelly" stools are associated with
    a. intussusception
    b. hemorrhoids
    c. Crohn's disease
    d. irritable bowel syndrome

165. The mortality rate for shaken baby syndrome is closest to
    a. 15%
    b. 30%
    c. 40%
    d. 50%

166. A patient arrives by ambulance after a fight. The patient has Battle's sign, clear fluid leaking from his ear, and his face feels boggy. You suspect:
    a. a frontal lobe contusion
    b. a basilar skull fracture
    c. pancreatitis
    d. appendicitis

167. You are caring for a patient who just arrived with a head injury. CT scan shows an epidural hematoma. You know this is an emergency because which artery has been torn?
    a. vertebral artery
    b. anterior cerebral artery
    c. middle cerebral artery
    d. middle meningeal artery

168. A 33-year-old man fell off a bicycle and sustained facial trauma. He complains of pain over the left cheek. Plain radiographs of the facial bones reveal an air–fluid level in the left maxillary sinus. What clinical condition should the nurse be most alert for?
    a. sinus infection
    b. excessive blood loss
    c. extraocular muscle entrapment
    d. anosmia

169. All of the following hormones are produced by the anterior pituitary EXCEPT
    a. adrenocorticotropic hormone (ACTH)
    b. prolactin
    c. oxytocin
    d. growth hormone

170. In treating diabetic ketoacidosis (DKA), dextrose is added to the IV fluids when the blood glucose level reaches
    a. 80 to 100 mg/dL
    b. 150 to 200 mg/dL
    c. 250 to 300 mg/dL
    d. 350 mg/dL

171. You are caring for a patient who just arrived in the ED from a long term care facility. The patient has fever, cloudy urine, and flank pain. Which one of the following types of urinary stones is associated with chronic urinary tract infections?
    a. uric acid
    b. calcium oxalate
    c. cystine
    d. struvite

172. Which of the following drugs is NOT effective when given endotracheally in a resuscitation situation?
    a. epinephrine
    b. lidocaine
    c. sodium bicarbonate
    d. naloxone

173. Risk factors for sudden infant death syndrome (SIDS) include all of the following EXCEPT
    a. infant siblings of a SIDS infant
    b. low-birth-weight preterm infants
    c. infants who sleep in a supine position
    d. infants who sleep in a prone position

174. Which of the following is not characteristic of atrial fibrillation?
    a. thrombus formation
    b. normal QRS complexes
    c. irregular pulse
    d. atrial rate of 120 per minute

175. A greenstick fracture
    a. is a type of pathologic fracture.
    b. is a fracture only on one side of the shaft of a bone.
    c. is present when fractured bone is exposed outside the skin.
    d. is characterized by a spiral break on a bone.

Answer Key and Explanations

1. B: All of the above actions may be appropriate depending on her situation; however, assessing her for suicidal ideation is your priority. If the patient is not suicidal, giving her a prescription for an antidepressant and recommending psychological counseling are essential. If the patient is suicidal, then admission may be the appropriate next step, especially if the patient has a plan and is a danger to herself or others. The admitting psychiatrist should be contacted to assess the patient as well.

2. C: Panic attacks are brief episodes of severe fear and anxiety that can manifest in a physical manner. Patients often feel as if they are dying and their symptoms can mimic those of a heart attack. A cardiac workup can sometimes be necessary to rule out a physical reason for their symptoms. Patients may experience hyperventilation, palpitations, racing heart rate, chest pain and pressure, and dizziness. Diarrhea is not a symptom of an acute panic attack, though nausea and vomiting are. Treatment in the ED may include anxiolytics, such as diazepam or lorazepam. Further psychiatric evaluation may be in order if the symptoms reoccur or if fear of another attack begins to interfere with the patient's daily life.

3. C: When treating a patient who has been brought in by the police, the handcuffs should not be removed, even if he is calm. Instead, you can offer a bedpan if he needs to use the bathroom. Using haloperidol in this manner can be considered a chemical restraint and may not be appropriate, unless he becomes violent or dangerous again. Anyone who has been violent or brought in by the police should not be discharged against medical advice because of the possibility of the patient harming himself or others. Additionally, charges may be brought against the patient so he must remain in the police custody. Providing the psychiatric patient with a private room with a minimal amount of stimulation can help him remain calm and minimize the risk for violence.

4. D: Naloxone is used to treat an overdose of opiates, such as heroin or morphine. Flumazenil is used as an antidote to benzodiazepines, including diazepam, lorazepam, or alprazolam. Diazepam cannot be used to treat an acute *Tylenol* overdose. N-acetylcysteine is the only drug that can neutralize the hepatotoxic metabolites that form with the excessive ingestion of acetaminophen.

5. A: Patients with bulimia tend to go through cycles of binging and purging, in which they eat large amounts of food and then engage in behaviors such as fasting, vomiting, or laxative abuse in an attempt to compensate. Patients with bulimia can often maintain a normal weight and do not typically have the emaciated appearance that patients with anorexia do. Dental carries or the loss of enamel is common because their teeth are frequently exposed to gastric acids during vomiting. Frequent induction of vomiting can also cause the knuckles to be scarred if they come into contact with the teeth. Electrolyte imbalances are common in patients with anorexia or bulimia.

6. B: These are all symptoms of a possible ectopic pregnancy. An immediate progesterone and pregnancy blood test should be ordered to confirm (or deny) the presence of a pregnancy, even if the patient denies being sexually active. A positive pregnancy test, low

progesterone level, and the absence of an intrauterine gestational sac on ultrasound are all indicators of an ectopic pregnancy. Rho(D) immune globulin may be necessary, but only if the patient is RH negative. Methotrexate will be given to disrupt and inhibit further growth of the pregnancy if it has not ruptured and is still small enough (less than 3.5 cm). It is not appropriate to administer magnesium sulfate or oxytocin in the case of an ectopic pregnancy.

7. C: First, convert the baby's weight in pounds to kilograms. 1 kg is equal to 2.2 lb, so divide 2 by 2.2, giving you 0.9 kg. Then, multiply the ordered dose of medication by the weight in kilograms to get 0.18 mL.

8. D: When a laboring patient has a prolapsed cord, an emergency cesarean delivery is indicated. Placing the patient in the Trendelenburg position (with her feet elevated and head dropped) will cause gravity to assist in relieving some of the pressure on the cord. Inserting a gloved hand into the vagina and applying manual pressure to the presenting part of the baby can also be extremely helpful. Administering extra oxygen and monitoring the fetal heart rate are also necessary. Placing the patient on her right side has no benefit.

9. D: When the victim of a rape or sexual assault is being treated, all of the above should be collected within 72 hours as part of a forensic rape kit. Questioning of the patient should include what happened, when, how, and by whom. Although it may be uncomfortable for the victim to answer, the more details that the nurse can elicit, the more helpful they will be. Great sensitivity should be used when speaking with a victim of sexual assault. In addition, samples from inside the mouth, rectum, vagina, and under the fingernails should be taken for possible DNA evidence. Finally, photographs of any bruising, lacerations, or other injuries should be taken and included with the kit as well. They may help identify a weapon or the assailant.

10. B: When testing with nitrazine paper indicates a pH greater then 4.5, a bacterial vaginal infection or *Trichomonas* infection is the most common cause. A combination of clindamycin and metronidazole will treat both bacterial and trichomonal infections. Clindamycin 2% should be applied vaginally at bedtime for 7 days. Metronidazole 500 mg should be taken by mouth twice a day for 7 days and a 0.75% cream should be applied intravaginally twice daily for 5 days. Fluconazole and antifungal creams are appropriate for fungal or yeast infections. Hydrocortisone cream can be appropriate in cases of an allergic external vaginitis, and should not be used internally.

11. A: Patients with small kidney stones in whom there is no concurrent infection will not have a fever. Flank pain and hematuria are symptoms common in both pyelonephritis and kidney stones. Diaphoresis is also a sign of kidney or urinary stones. Renal calculi occur most often in men and are associated with certain medical conditions or lifestyle factors. They are most often composed of calcium.

12. A: Irrigating the bladder when not a part of the patient's medical care plan increases the risk of introducing bacteria into the urinary tract. Utilizing a closed drainage system with an indwelling catheter can decrease that risk and should always be used when possible. Aseptic technique and gently cleaning the urinary meatus can also reduce the risk for infection. Other techniques include minimizing their use when possible, not placing catheterized patients in close proximity to infectious patients, and maintaining proper urinary drainage and flow.

13. C: Acute prostatitis is an infection of the prostate gland, usually due to *E. coli* or *S. aureus*. Symptoms include fever and chills, low back or perineal pain, and painful urination or urinary frequency. Incontinence is not a sign of acute prostatitis, but can indicate other prostate problems, such as benign prostatic hypertrophy or hyperplasia. Treatment of choice for prostatitis is ciprofloxacin 500 mg orally twice daily for 1 month.

14. D: The correct antidote of benzodiazepine toxicity is to administer flumazenil 0.2 mg each minute up to 3 mg total. However, flumazenil should never be given in a patient with increased intracranial pressure, making frequent monitoring essential. Supportive respiratory care may become necessary also because respiratory depression can sometimes occur. Charcoal can help bind toxic substances in the GI tract and is not contraindicated in benzodiazepine intoxication. Fomepizole is the antidote for ethylene glycol toxicity (antifreeze ingestion).

15. A: Levofloxacin 500 mg orally once daily is the preferred treatment protocol for *Salmonella* infection. Antibiotics are needed in patients who are severely ill or immunocompromised, but can be withheld in a patient who is immunocompetent and only mildly ill. Symptoms of *Salmonella* infection include abdominal pain, fever, vomiting, and bloody diarrhea, and usually begin 1 to 3 days after infection. *Salmonella* bacteria are found in unpasteurized milk and dairy products, contaminated eggs, and undercooked meats.

16. B: Patient should be on her left side, with her head below her body. This prevents gastric contents from being emptied into the small intestine. Seated or other positions in which the head is elevated can also encourage gastric emptying. A patient can be put in the supine position if he has been intubated. Trendelenburg positioning has no benefit and may increase the risk for aspiration.

17. A, C, D, F: Per the "Rule of Nines," this patient has third-degree burns covering a total body surface area (BSA) of approximately 45% (9% for his head/neck, 9% for each arm, 18% for the front trunk). With such severe burns, the patient is at risk for severe electrolyte imbalances as the exposed tissue begins to experience fluid loss. Loss of calcium, sodium, and phosphorus, and increased potassium levels are the most common and dangerous imbalances. Monitoring for these imbalances and supplementing as necessary are priorities in treating patients with severe burns.

18. B: A patient with acute alcohol intoxication who is easily arousable and with normal vital signs can safely sleep off his intoxication. Endotracheal intubation is not necessary, unless his condition deteriorates. Gastric lavage will not be helpful because it has likely been more than 1 hour since the patient ingested alcohol. Discharging the patient is not appropriate given his disorientation and altered mental status, and the possibility of him hurting himself. The nurse should, however, check on the patient frequently and make sure that his neurological status does not change as time goes on.

19. A: Opening and debriding hemorrhagic blisters should be avoided in order to reduce the risk for infection. Debriding clear blisters can help prevent tissue damage as a result of exposure to prostaglandins and thromboxanes, which are released during inflammation. Aloe vera cream should be applied both to hemorrhagic and debrided clear blisters, and can also help minimize thromboxane exposure. Rapid rewarming is essential and should be performed as soon as possible, and when the risk of refreezing has been eliminated.

20. D: The classic bull's eye rash, joint pain, and flu-like symptoms, including headache, fatigue, stiff neck, and fever, are all common and early symptoms of Lyme disease. As the disease progresses, patients may also experience more profound joint pain and arthritis, confusion, memory loss, and numbness. Diarrhea is not a symptom of Lyme disease. Once the diagnosis has been confirmed, doxycycline or amoxicillin are the antibiotics of choice. Intravenous antibiotics may be indicated in more severe cases.

21. C: Deferoxamine is used to treat severe iron intoxication. Gastric lavage may also be helpful if the child swallowed the pills generally no longer than 1 hour prior. Flumazenil is used to treat benzodiazepine overdose; naloxone, an opiate overdose; and N-acetylcysteine, an acetaminophen overdose.

22. A: Using the trauma scoring system, he receives 2 points for a respiratory rate between 6 and 9 (4 points for 10 to 29 bpm, 3 points for more than 29 bpm, 1 point for 1 to 5 bpm, 0 points for not breathing). He scores 3 points for having a systolic blood pressure between 76 and 89 mm Hg (4 points for more than 89.3 mm Hg, 2 points for 40 to 75 mm Hg, 1 point for 1 to 39 mm Hg, 0 points for having no blood pressure). Finally, his GCS is 14, awarding him 4 points (3 points for GCS of 9 to 12, 2 points for GCS of 6 to 8, 1 point for GCS of 4 to 5, 0 points for GCS of 2). Adding up the assigned points (2 for respiratory, 3 for blood pressure, and 4 for GCS) gives the patient a score of 9.

23. B: The proximal tibia is the preferred site for intraosseous infusion in the pediatric patient, 5 years of age and younger. The medial malleolus, sternum, clavicle, humerus, ilium, and femur can all support intraosseous infusion in the adult or older pediatric patient, though intraosseous infusion is more difficult. A specially designed 13- to 20-gauge needle loaded into a bone insertion gun is needed to gain access. Correct positioning should be confirmed by withdrawing 5 mL of blood and bone marrow before using the site for infusion.

24. C: The patient is likely suffering from an anaphylactic reaction in response to something eaten at lunch. Albuterol 2.5 mg should be given to relieve the bronchospasm. Oxygen and fluids should also be administered for hypotension. Diphenhydramine should be administered to treat the underlying allergy, and methylprednisolone can be given if there is no relief with diphenhydramine. Frequent monitoring is necessary because of the potential for airway loss if the allergic reaction progresses. If that should happen, intubation may become necessary.

25. B: When a patient goes into shock, regardless of the cause, symptoms include hypotension, tachycardia, decreased urinary output, changes in respiratory pattern (either tachypnea or bradypnea), hypoxemia, and changed mental status. Lowered blood pressure reduces tissue perfusion. This means that there is less oxygen being delivered, and fewer waste products being removed from, the body tissues, causing cellular and tissue damage. Hypertension does not occur in any type of shock.

26. C: Classification of hypovolemic shock is based on the amount of fluid lost. Class I is appropriate when 750 mL or less (or 15% or less of total circulating volume) is lost. Class II is classified when there is a loss of 750 to 1,000 mL (15% to 30% blood volume loss). When 1,500 to 2,000 mL of fluid is lost (30% to 40% blood volume loss), it is classified as class III. Class IV occurs when more than 2,000 mL (or more than 40% blood volume loss) of fluid is lost. Hypovolemic shock can occur for a number of reasons, and is diagnosed when large

amounts of fluid are lost from the intravascular system. Common causes include blood loss, severe diarrhea or vomiting, internal fluid shifts, or a severe injury in which the integrity of large blood vessels is compromised.

27. B: The description of the hemodynamics point to distributive shock, which occurs when there is sufficient blood volume, but an underlying condition causes the vasculature to abnormally dilate. This reduces the ability of the vessels to effectively move the blood, leading to hypoperfusion. Neurogenic shock can lead to changes in vascular tone. As this patient was found after a fall you would suspect neurogenic shock, which is a type of distributive shock. Distributive shock may result from anaphylactic shock, septic shock, neurogenic shock, and drug ingestions.

28. B: Autotransfusion in the absence of donor blood is a great alternative, with few complications. Using a commercial kit is not necessary. In the case of a hemopneumothorax, blood can be collected directly into a sterile chest tube container, then IV tubing attached for transfusion. Heparinization is not necessary, though citrate phosphate dextrose is often added to the collected blood. Autotransfusion is contraindicated in cases in which the wound is more than 6 hours old, where the patient has a malignant tumor at the site of collection, or where obvious contamination of the wound has occurred.

29. A: A patient in septic shock may experience a multitude of systemic complications, including liver and renal failure. Patients in acute renal failure have elevated BUN levels and decreased urinary output. A patient in liver failure would have increased bilirubin and liver enzymes, not decreased. Lactic acid is increased, not decreased when a patient is in septic shock due to excess lactic acid production in times of tissue hypoperfusion. Hemodynamic changes can cause platelet levels to decrease, not increase.

30. D: Dopamine is a potent vasopressor and the drug of choice given to correct hypotension. It is administered IV at a rate of 0.5 to 5 mcg/kg/min. Dobutamine increases cardiac output and contractility, and is administered at a rate of 2 to 20 mcg/kg/min. Systolic blood pressure may or may not increase as a result of the increased cardiac output. Atropine is an antiarrhythmic used to treat bradycardia and is not used in the treatment of hypotension. Epinephrine is also a vasopressor, but is indicated in the treatment of cardiac arrest.

31. B: Blumberg sign is a symptom of peritonitis and is elicited when pain results from the depression and then rapid release of the abdominal cavity, also known as rebound tenderness. The psoas and obturator signs indicate irritation of the appendix and are elicited when the hips are flexed and internally rotated (the obturator sign) or when the right hip is passively extended by the examiner as the patient is laying on her left side (the psoas sign). Currant jelly stool, or stool that is composed of blood and mucus, is seen in patients with intussusception of the intestines.

32. B: Metronidazole for 1 week to 10 days is the preferred antibiotic for treating a *C. difficile* infection, though vancomycin may also be used. Symptoms of *C. difficile* infection often occur after antibiotic use and include bloody diarrhea and abdominal pain. Clindamycin is not used to treat *C. difficile* infection, and in fact is often the antibiotic culprit indicated in disrupting normal colonic flora, causing *C. diff*. One of the standards of treatment is stopping the inciting antibiotic and starting the patient on a new one if needed. Patients are put on contact precautions and must be educated regarding using actual hand

rubbing with soap and water to remove the spores of C. *difficile* to prevent spreading the infection.

33. D: GERD is the chronic regurgitation of stomach acids into the esophagus, causing cellular and tissue damage over the long-term, including Barrett esophagus and esophageal cancer. Symptoms of a peptic ulcer include bloody/tarry stools, nausea, vomiting, and abdominal pain, and occur when an overproduction of stomach acid irritates the lining of the GI tract. Cholecystitis is the inflammation and obstruction of the bile duct, and most commonly occurs in women who are overweight and between 20 to 40 years of age. Severe upper right quadrant pain, sometimes radiating to the back, and nausea/vomiting are the most common symptoms. Patients with pancreatitis also present with abdominal pain and nausea/vomiting. Their pain is often in the left upper quadrant.

34. A: The symptoms indicate that this child likely has intussusceptions, a condition where the intestines telescope into one another. In addition to the above symptoms, many children also pass stool that resembles currant jelly (filled with blood and mucus). Early identification and treatment are keys to preventing necrosis of the intestinal tissue. A barium or air enema may provide enough pressure to resolve the intussusception, but surgery may become necessary if complications begin to develop or the enema is not effective. A child with appendicitis or constipation would not have the sausage-shaped mass but may have signs of abdominal pain. A child with a hernia may also have severe abdominal pain and a small soft mass in the belly, but may also have other signs such as tachycardia and nausea/vomiting.

35. C: Bruising around the umbilicus, Cullen sign, is the most common signs of splenic rupture. Left shoulder pain, or Kehr sign, is frequently seen in patients with intra-abdominal bleeding. Splenic injuries occur frequently in blunt abdominal trauma simply because the spleen is not as well protected by the ribs as other organs. In contrast, pancreatic injuries are less common from blunt trauma because the pancreas is so well protected. Patients with pancreatic injuries may also vomit bile, in addition to having diffuse abdominal pain. Intestinal perforation is significantly more likely to occur with penetrating trauma, such as a gunshot or knife wound, than with blunt trauma from a motor vehicle accident. Symptoms include acute abdominal pain, distention and rigidity, tachycardia, and nausea/vomiting.

36. A: FAST (focused assessment with sonography for trauma) is a rapid ultrasound performed at the bedside when abdominal or pericardial injury is suspected. In the emergency room setting, only a physician with sufficient training in sonography should perform the sonogram. The physician will quickly assess all 4 quadrants of the abdomen and the pericardium to look for free fluid or other evidence of bleeding.

37. B: In order to properly estimate the NG tube insertion length, measure the distance (in centimeters) from the patient's earlobe to the xiphoid process, and the distance from the patient's earlobe to the tip of her nose. Add these two distances together and add on an additional 15 cm. If possible, the patient should be seated upright and swallow small sips of water as you pass the tube through the nares. This should help the patient comfortably swallow the tube into the esophagus. A topical anesthetic in the throat can help reduce the gag reflex. Placement of the tube should be confirmed with an x-ray.

38. D: All of the symptoms listed in the question are signs of epiglottitis. A child with acute tracheitis will have the same "croupy" or barky cough, but with a high fever and copious

amounts of thick tracheal secretions, which have the potential to obstruct the airway. A patient with a peritonsillar abscess will have similar symptoms to epiglottitis, including fever and hoarseness of the voice, but will also have swelling and redness of the tonsils and possibly the palate. A patient with epiglottitis requires close observation because of the potential rapid progression to complete airway obstruction.

39. B: Temporal arteritis occurs when the large blood vessels in the head, especially the temporal artery and branches of the thoracic aorta, become inflamed. This is most commonly seen in adults older than 50 years of age and is sometimes associated with other immunodeficiencies. Symptoms include headaches, fever, visual changes, and pain in the jaw and tongue. If diagnosis of this syndrome is suspected, treatment with prednisone 60 mg daily should begin immediately to prevent the progression to blindness. A definitive diagnosis is made with a temporal artery biopsy.

40. B: NSAIDS should be avoided in the patient with a hyphema, Tylenol is a good choice for pain relief. The other interventions are appropriate and standards of care. A hyphema is the building up of blood in the anterior chamber of the eye and is usually caused by a trauma of some sort. Grade 1 hyphema is when the accumulating blood occupies less than a third of the anterior chamber. Grade 2 hyphema is when the accumulating blood occupies between one-third and one-half of the chamber; grade 3, more than half of the chamber; grade 4, the entire anterior chamber of the eye.

41. D: A tooth avulsion is a complete removal of the tooth from the socket. Permanent teeth can be reimplanted within an hour or two of the avulsion. The tooth should be transported from the scene of the accident in either milk or saline. The tooth should be cleaned with either saline of Hanks solution, taking care to not handle any of the remaining nerve fibers. They should not be trimmed or disrupted in any way. If the tooth has dried out and it has been less than an hour, the tooth should be soaked in Hanks solution for approximately 30 minutes before it can be reimplanted. If the tooth has been dried out for more than an hour, it should go through a series of solutions to prepare it: citric acid for 5 minutes, stannous fluoride 2% for 5 minutes, and finally doxycycline solution for 5 minutes. To reimplant the tooth, the socket should be gently cleaned and the tooth placed firmly in place, with a piece of gauze covering it. The patient should bite down firmly while a splint is applied directly to the affected tooth and the 4 teeth surrounding it.

42. A: Eye pain is not a symptom of retinal detachment. Patients experience painless changes in vision, such as the loss of central vision, seeing floaters or cobwebs in the field of vision, and appearances of flashes of light (photopsia). If retinal detachment is confirmed during a fundal exam, the patient should be referred to a retinal surgeon for the repair.

43. B: All of these are important measures of a thorough and well-executed research study. Internal validity is when a study has confirmed a cause-and-effect relationship between two variables without any interference coming between the two variables. The cause must come before the effect. External validity is when the results found during the study apply to other environments, populations, and groups. Sample size and selection are important factors when evaluating the results as well. The sample group must be large enough and diverse enough, or the study may not hold true.

44. D: The focus during the incident is to treat patients and manage the immediate crisis situation. However, once the situation has been resolved, there should be a group meeting

to review the incident and educate the staff about posttraumatic stress and the resources that are available to them. Mental health care professionals should be accessible and the staff should also be given pamphlets, handouts, and educational materials about getting additional support. The staff should also be educated about how they can support each other during that time.

45. A: The nurse should only delegate tasks that the technician is qualified to handle. It is important to remember that the nurse remains responsible for all delegated tasks. Unlicensed personnel should never be responsible for assessing a patient, an essential skill when checking on a patient after his first dose of an opiate. Transporting an unstable patient should only be the responsibility of a physician or other practitioner who is able to manage the patient should his condition deteriorate. Changing wound dressings are part of a nurse's responsibility; nurses should assess the wound and administer ordered medications or treatments in addition to changing the bandages. Unlicensed personnel can often assist a patient to the restroom if the patient is stable and could alert the nurse if his or her assistance is needed for the given situation.

46. C: Reporting responsibilities are a matter of law, not personal opinion or patient confidentiality. For that reason, the nurse must report the diagnosis according to the state and federal guidelines. The nurse should inform the patient of her responsibilities and why guidelines must be followed.

47. D: Given the ethical implications of this case, it should certainly be brought to the doctor's attention, as well as your nursing supervisor. Assembling an ethics committee may be warranted, and the nursing supervisor will be able to assist and possibly serve on the committee. Nothing should be done until the hospital's policies and ethical standards are investigated. The family should be informed about the process so that they can be involved in the process and assist if necessary.

48. B: While calling the police may be mandatory depending on the state in which you live, you should assess the patient and her actual risk for abuse before contacting the authorities. First, ask the boyfriend to step out of the room and ask the patient (in a sensitive manner) about how her injury and bruises occurred. There may be an alternate and reasonable cause for her injuries. If you still believe that she is being abused, you can provide further information about creating a safety or escape plan, and even recommend that she speak with the social worker. Regardless of whether she admits to being abused or not, her injuries should be treated. Alternate discharge placement can also be arranged if she wishes.

49. D: A patient with increased intracranial pressure should be placed in the supine position, with the head of the bed elevated 30 degrees to promote drainage of excess fluid. Medications may be necessary, not only to keep a patient pain free, but also to prevent agitation. Use of diuretics can also help reduce extra fluid in the brain. Mechanical ventilation or other respiratory support should be provided if the patient is unable to breathe sufficiently on his own. Additionally, the patient's electrolytes should be monitored closely in case fluid or electrolyte replacement is needed.

50. C: Upon assessment of the patient, you can assign a score of 2 points for eye movement (4, spontaneous eye opening; 3, eyes opening in response to verbal stimuli; 2, eyes opening in response to painful stimuli; 1, no eye opening). The patient is assigned a score of 1 for

verbal response (5, alert and oriented; 4, alert but confused; 3, not able to appropriately answer questions or uses inappropriate language; 2, speech is unintelligible; 1, patient is not responsive). Finally, the patient is assigned a score of 4 for motor response (6, patient is able to obey commands; 5, moves in a purposeful manner in response to pain; 4, withdraws from pain; 3, decorticate posturing or abnormal flexion to pain; 2, decerebrate posturing or abnormal extension to pain; 1, no response to pain). Two plus one plus four gives a score of 7.

51. D: Measures to decrease intracranial pressure include: Elevating the head of the bed 30 degrees to promote drainage, keeping head midline, oral intubation instead of nasotracheal if ventilation required, analgesia to control pain and reduce agitation, sedation: propofol (adults only), benzodiazepines, respiratory support, including ventilation with oxygen administration to increase perfusion, hyperventilation is used only if herniation of the brain is imminent, drainage of cerebrospinal fluid as indicated, diuretics, induction of coma with pentobarbital, and volume replacement. This patient does not have signs of herniating.

52. B: Giving antihypertensives and anti-seizure medication is standard treatment. Patients need to be monitored closely for sign of neurological deterioration that could indicate re-bleeding. Subarachnoid hemorrhage is graded according to the following: Grade I: No symptoms or slight headache and nuchal rigidity, Grade II: Mod-severe headache with nuchal rigidity and cranial nerve palsy, Grade III: Drowsy, progressing to confusion or mild focal deficits, Grade IV: Stupor, with hemiparesis (mod-severe), early decerebrate rigidity, and vegetative disturbances, and Grade V: Coma state with decerebrate rigidity. The scenario does not mention the patient having any respiratory distress, and is obviously alert enough to report pain so immediate intubation would not be warranted at this time.

53. C: In a tonic-clonic seizure (also called grand mal seizure), a patient initially has stiffening over the entire body. Her eyes may roll back in her head and she may lose consciousness. This is called the tonic period and lasts anywhere between 10 and 30 seconds. Following the tonic period is the clonic period of the seizure, again lasting around 30 seconds. The patient suffers violent and rhythmic contractions over her whole body. The patient may lose continence of both urine and feces. After the seizure is over, the patient often experiences confusion, disorientation, and n/v. They may fall asleep and waken conscious.

54. A: The cauda equina ("horse's tail") is the lower, ending portion of the spinal cord. Symptoms of damage to this part of the spinal cord include incontinence and varying degrees of paralysis or loss of sensation to the lower extremities. Damage to the central cord would produce quadriparesis, worsening in degree according to how superior the injury is. Posterior cord damage would produce deficits in sensation but the patient would likely retain his motor skills. A patient with anterior cord damage would be completely paralyzed, but the sensations of touch and vibration would most likely not be affected.

55. C: Administration of corticosteroids should begin within 8 hours after the injury occurred. Methylprednisolone 30 mg/kg should be given as an IV bolus (over approximately 15 minutes). Once the initial bolus has been administered, the patient should be given a 45-minute break, and then a methylprednisolone drip should be started at a rate of 5.4 mg/kg per hour for 23 hours.

56. B: Namenda and dextromethorphan, a common ingredient found in nonprescription cough syrups, both work in the exact same way and should not be used together because of the potential for adverse effects. They inhibit certain chemicals in the brain that regulate glutamate activity.

57. A: Multiple sclerosis is an autoimmune disorder that is most commonly diagnosed in younger adults in their 20s. Symptoms vary widely and can also include bladder dysfunction, pain, and tremors. Myasthenia gravis is also an autoimmune disorder that can produce speech and visual abnormalities, but balance and coordination would not be affected. Given that the patient has been living with these symptoms for so long, it is unlikely that she has had a stroke. Patients with ALS would not have visual disturbances.

58. D: tPA should not be administered to anyone who has a recent history of a stroke, surgery, or other hemorrhagic incident. tPA is also contraindicated in patients with a low platelet count (ie, below 100,000 cells/cu mm). Anticoagulation therapy should be initiated within 3 hours. Patients with uncontrolled blood pressure should not be given tPA because of the potential for hypertensive episodes. However, antihypertensives can supplement administration of tPA in a patient who has well-controlled and mild hypertension.

59. D: Nuchal rigidity is a stiffness of the neck and can indicate irritation of the covering of the brain or spinal cord. The test is positive usually in cases of meningitis. To assess for this sign, the nurse should place her hands behind the patient's head and slightly flex the head forward. The test is considered positive if the maneuver causes pain or increased resistance. Nuchal rigidity is a symptom of bacterial meningitis, subarachnoid hemorrhage, and leukemia.

60. D: Seizures, hypertension, and peptic ulcers are relative contraindications but are not absolute contraindications. This patient has significant respiratory and neurologic symptoms, and the physician has decided that the benefits for this patient outweigh the risks. The nurse should notify the physician of the daughter's questions.

61. D: People have very different experiences of pain and have varying behaviors associated with it. Some people cry and show a lot of physical symptoms with very little pain, while on the other end of the spectrum, some people do not show any physical signs of discomfort even with excruciating pain. For that reason, you have to trust the assessment that the patient is making of her own pain and not involve your judgment of the situation. As part of your assessment, however, you should elicit more information about the quality of her pain and document that as well.

62. C: Unstable patients or women in active labor should not be transferred out of the ED until the clinical situation has stabilized (or the baby was delivered). If necessary, an obstetrician can come down to the ED to assist during the delivery if the ED physician is concerned about complications. Assuming that the hospital is able to care for the newborn, there would be no reason to consider transferring the patient or her baby off premises, so the woman (and her baby) should be brought to the postpartum and nursery departments to recover.

63. B: The patient has injuries that definitely need to be treated, but can wait until after the more severe and life-threatening injuries have been handled. She should be periodically assessed for blood loss from the amputation site to make sure that her status has not changed.

64. A: Whenever you are uncertain about a medication order, you should clarify the order with the physician and even your written orders (either on the computer or in the paper chart). Perhaps he changed his mind on a dose or drug and forgot to notify you of the change. Once you have confirmed that a mistake was made, notify the pharmacy immediately so that the correct medication can be sent to your unit.

65. D: You should never apply restraints, either chemical or physical, unless there are absolutely no other alternatives or you are concerned about the patient hurting herself or others. There is a very real concern that the patient may wander off the unit, so simply checking on her frequently is not appropriate, especially if you get caught up in another more medically pressing emergency. Assigning someone to sit with and keep an eye on her is the best course of action in this case.

66. A: First, you must convert the patient's weight to kilograms by dividing 120 by 2.2. The patient weighs 54.5 kg. Multiply by the ordered dose (10 mg/kg) to determine how much should be administered, which is 545 mg. Divide by the rate (45 mg/min) to determine the number of minutes for the infusion, or 12 minutes.

67. A and C: The 5 rights of medication administration are right patient, right dose, right drug, right timing and frequency, and right route of administration. The order in which the medications are administered is not included.

68. A: When changing a dressing, only gloves are needed, unless the patient is under isolation precautions. You would also don a gown and mask if you were concerned about the splattering of blood or body fluids, which may pose a risk for contamination of your clothing or eyes, nose, or mouth.

69. B: The optimal temperature for an amputated part before reattachment is 4°C. The amputated limb should be reattached within 6 hours, but if well cared for, that time can be extended up to 24 hours. Any jewelry remaining on the limb should be removed. The limb should be washed thoroughly in normal saline, and then wrapped in a moist dressing. To cool the limb, place in a plastic bag, then immerse the sealed bag in a solution of ice water. Check it frequently to make sure that the part has not frozen.

70. C: You should never squeeze the stinger while it is still in the skin because it will release more venom into the skin and worsen the reaction. Gently scrape a sharp instrument over the area until the stinger comes out. You can apply ice afterwards to reduce swelling and as a comfort measure. Apply the ice pack for 10 to 20 minutes, and then take off for 10 to 20 minutes for up to 24 hours.

71. C: After a tick bite, the tick should be removed and sealed in a dated plastic bag. Place in the freezer for a few weeks until the patient shows no evidence of illness. The patient should also be counseled to report any flu-like symptoms or suspicious rashes with the "bull's eye" shape.

72. D: Compartment syndrome occurs after an injury, when swelling or bleeding into the muscle compartment cuts off blood flow to the muscle tissue. Symptoms include numbness, tingling, cyanosis, and swelling of the affected limb. Patients often have decreased pulses in the distal arteries and severe pain unrelieved by pain medication.

73. A: The Tinel test is performed when the examiner gently taps or percusses over the medial nerve of the affected wrist. A positive result is when the maneuver causes pain or numbness and is indicative of carpal tunnel syndrome, compression of the median nerve in the wrist. It is most commonly associated with pregnancy, repetitive hand motions such as typing, arthritis, and diabetes. The other test used to diagnose carpal tunnel is the Phalen test, where both wrists are flexed and the back of the hands are touching. If positive, this position will also cause pain or numbness.

74. C: Treatment protocols for dislocation and fracture include reduction of the affected area, immobilization using a cast, brace, or sling, and cold compresses to reduce swelling. Application of heat is not an appropriate intervention. Referral to an orthopedic specialist may be necessary if complications are present or the dislocation is not able to be reduced in the ED.

75. C: *Neisseria gonorrhoeae* is the strain of bacteria most commonly associated with infectious arthritis. Other implicated bacteria include *Streptococcus*, *Staphylococcus*, and *E. coli*. Rubella does cause infectious arthritis but is a virus, not a bacterium. Other viral causes include hepatitis B and parvovirus. Certain fungi and parasites can also cause infectious arthritis.

76. B: Gout is a condition in which high serum levels of uric acid can cause crystals to deposit in the joints and cause pain and inflammation. A uric acid blood level above 7 mg/dL indicates that the patient may have gout. Treatment includes reducing consumption of foods high in purines, such as alcohol and organ meats, NSAIDs for pain relief, and probenecid or allopurinol to prevent formation of the uric acid crystals over the long term.

77. C: For a simple muscle strain or sprain, ice should be applied to the affected area for the first 48 hours. The injury should also be rested and elevated. After the first 48 hours has passed, heat should be applied for 15 to 20 minutes, several times each day.

78. D: To measure venous refill, have the patient lie in the supine position for a few minutes, then have the patient sit up with her feet dangling. Watch for filling of the veins on the feet and count the time. If it takes longer than 20 seconds for the veins to regain their normal full state, a possible venous occlusion is indicated.

79. B: Normal pulse intensity is documented as 2. The remainder of the scale is as follows:
>   0 – Absent pulses
>   1 – Weak or thready pulse
>   2 – Normal
>   3 – Full pulse
>   4 – Bounding pulse

In addition to measuring the intensity of a patient's pulse, the rate and rhythm should be assessed and documented. If one of the parameters is abnormal, further evaluation may be necessary, such as checking the pulse bilaterally, further distally or proximally, or with positional changes.

80. A: Patients with measles should be placed in a room with negative air pressure to prevent transmission of the infection. Caregivers should always wear a mask, gown, and gloves when providing care, and the patient should also wear a mask and clean gown when

- 42 -

outside of the room. Nurses and other caregivers should also wear a mask, gown, and gloves when caring for the patient with pertussis, influenza, and pneumonia, but the patient does not need to be confined to a room with negative air pressure.

81. C: A patient in DIC has the conflicting conditions of both hemorrhage and coagulation at the same time. Tissue factor enters the bloodstream and binds with various coagulation factors. Fibrinogen is converted to fibrin by thrombin; therefore, you would expect to see a decrease in fibrinogen levels. This then causes the platelets to aggregate and eventually clot, again, decreasing platelet levels. As the clots get larger, they break off and enter the bloodstream, which can eventually cause blockages in small blood vessels. The formation of these clots results in the breakdown of fibrin and fibrinogen, leading to the destruction of the clots and subsequent hemorrhage.

82. B: All of these interventions are appropriate for this patient, but the most important one right now is to stop the bleeding, in this case begin by trying to pinch the nose and have the child lean forward. Patients with type A hemophilia are missing clotting factor VII, which is the most common type of hemophilia. Males are much more commonly affected because of the mode of inheritance; hemophilia is usually X-linked. Patients with type B hemophilia are missing factor IX, and patients lacking factor XI have type C. Type C hemophilia is quite rare in the United States and is equally diagnosed in both males and females.

83. D: It is likely this patient is presenting with pneumocystis pneumonia, and all these interventions are likely appropriate, but as the patient likely has pneumonia, antibiotics need to be started quickly (in at least 6 hours of presentation to the ER to meet Core Measures), this patient needs to have the blood cultures drawn first so that the antibiotics can be started. Because the prompt says that this patient has AIDS, and human immunodeficiency virus (HIV) has officially progressed to acquired immunodeficiency syndrome once CD4 counts are below 200 cells/mm^3, as well as the presence of a defining condition, such as Kaposi sarcoma, cytomegalovirus (CMV), or wasting syndrome, we know the CD4 count is low. CD4 counts should be checked periodically to determine the immune status of the patient, but it isn't priority right now.

84. D: A patient with HHNK would have an increased serum osmolality. The patient would also have a severely elevated blood glucose level and increased BUN and creatinine levels. HHNK most frequently occurs in people who may have a prolonged history of insulin resistance, but otherwise no other diagnosis of diabetes. Persistently elevated blood sugar levels can cause fluid to shift in the body to the extracellular spaces. This is an attempt to maintain osmotic equilibrium, but instead causes dehydration and electrolyte imbalances, increasing the blood osmolality.

85. B: Reed-Sternberg cells are B cells that are abnormal in size and shape. When present, they indicate that the patient most likely has Hodgkin lymphoma. Some of the physical signs (enlarged lymph nodes, fever, and weakness) would also be present in a patient with leukemia and even non-Hodgkin lymphoma. Reed-Sternberg cells are only found in Hodgkin lymphoma, distinguishing it from other lymphomas or blood cancers.

86. A: The normal WBC count for the average adult is 4,500 to 11,000/mm^3. However, a normal WBC in neonates is considerably higher, around 9,000 to 30,000/mm^3. As the child ages, what is considered to be a normal WBC count begins to decrease, between 5,000 to

around 20,000/mm³ by 1 month of age; 6,000 to 17,500/mm³ throughout toddlerhood; and just about the normal adult count by the teenage years.

87. C: A scabies infection is one caused by a small mite that has burrowed into the skin; the mite creates straight, raised "tracks" where they burrow. They are spread very easily and outbreaks are common in nursing homes or other long-term facilities. Treatment involves applying permethrin 5% cream over the entire body. The patient is then allowed to shower, removing the cream about 12 hours after application. A second treatment is prescribed in 1 week. Because the burrowing can cause extreme itching, antihistamines can also be prescribed. Griseofulvin is used to treat fungal infections, and niclosamide is used for tapeworms. Doxycycline may be necessary to treat skin infections caused when the patient scratches the skin to relieve the itching, but will not kill the mites.

88. A: A patient who has a small, painless chancre on his genitalia is in the primary phase of syphilis. This phase can last up to 3 to 6 weeks. Once the symptoms become systemic (ie, flu-like symptoms, headache, body aches, sore throat), the infection has progressed to the secondary stage. A patient may also have a red rash covering his trunk, hands, or feet. This will occur several weeks after the initial infection and may or may not resolve. Once the patient has neurological or cardiovascular symptoms, he is infected with tertiary, or latent, syphilis.

89. C: Doxycycline 100 mg orally twice daily or azithromycin 1 g orally x 1 dose are the preferred treatments for chlamydia. The patient should be recultured after completing the antibiotic regimen to ensure that the infection has been cured. It is also extremely important for the patient to contact relevant sexual partners and avoid sexual contact until the infection is gone. (This usually takes a week if recultures show antibiotic has been successful). The nurse will likely need to report the infection to the Board of Health once diagnosis has been confirmed.

90. D: Prior to accessing an AV fistula for hemodialysis, the skin should be washed with a povidone-iodine solution to minimize the risk for infection. The nurse should also auscultate the fistula to make sure that the line is patent and working properly. An AV fistula should never be used for any procedure other than hemodialysis or in the rare case of an extreme emergency when other venous sources cannot be accessed.

91. B: Febrile seizures are most common in young children, usually between the ages of 6 months and 5 years, and in situations in which a very high fever is involved. They usually are not serious, but the child should be evaluated to ensure that there is no underlying cause to the seizure. In the case of an uncomplicated seizure, the parents should administer acetaminophen as instructed and place the child in a tepid bath to help bring her temperature down.

92. A: First, convert the child's weight in pounds to kilograms by dividing by 2.2. This gives a weight of 7.3 kgs. Then, multiply by the dose (15 mg/kg) to determine how much medication the child should receive. 7.3 x 15 = 109 mg.

93. B: While the correct placement of an endotracheal tube should always be verified after insertion, a good guide is 21 cm for female patients and 23 cm for males. For children older than the age of 2, divide their age (in years) by 2 and add 12 cm. Therefore, for a 4-year-old child, divide 4 by 2 (your answer is 2) and add 12 cm. That gives you the proper insertion

depth of 14 cm. You can verify placement by using an end-tidal CO_2 detector, which attaches to the endotracheal tube and checks the concentration of CO_2 that is exhaled.

94. A: Normal values for the partial pressure of CO_2 are 35 to 45 mm Hg and for the partial pressure of oxygen are above 80 mm Hg. A patient in respiratory failure would have difficulty taking in oxygen and then subsequently removing the excess carbon dioxide. This would raise the $PaCO_2$ and lower the PaO_2, making choice A the correct one.

95. B: Chances are that the child or his/her parent already tried the rescue inhaler without success before bringing the child into the ED. Waiting to see if it worked may require precious minutes in which the child does not get any oxygen. Intubation is contraindicated in patients with status asthmaticus because the insertion of the tube can cause additional trauma and swelling to the already inflamed bronchi. Theophylline is also contraindicated in young children and should only be used in dire situations. Albuterol is a beta-adrenergic agonist, which relaxes bronchial smooth muscle tissue. It can be used alone or in conjunction with an anticholinergic, such as ipratropium.

96. D: *S. aureus* is the pathogen that most commonly causes acute tracheitis in young children. *H. influenzae* and group A *Streptococcus* can also occasionally cause tracheitis, though *S. aureus* is significantly more likely. In addition to the typical symptoms of a laryngobronchitis, patients produce large amounts of copious, thick tracheal discharge. Because of this, patients often need to be ventilated in order to maintain their airway as they fight the infection.

97. C: A patient has respiratory alkalosis when he excretes larger than normal amounts of CO_2. This reduces $PaCO_2$, which causes a decrease in the amount of carbonic acid (H_2CO_3) in the blood. The kidneys attempt to compensate by excreting HCO_3 and retaining extra hydrogen molecules. The extra hydrogen causes the pH to increase (creating the alkalosis environment). A decreased pH would not be observed in cases of respiratory alkalosis.

98. C: A patient with interstitial pneumonia has an infection affecting their alveoli or the interstitium. In interstitial pneumonia, the alveoli are destroyed as they fill with fluid or exudates. When the lobes of the lung (one or more) are affected, it is called lobar pneumonia. Bronchial or lobular pneumonia is the term given to infections of the lower or terminal ends of the bronchioles.

99. D: A tension pneumothorax is when a laceration to the pleural sac allows air to enter the pleural space but not be removed, causing a great deal of pressure in the sac. The mediastinum and trachea are often forced to shift in order to accommodate the extra pressure. Diagnostically, the clinician may also observe decreased breath sounds and acute pain on the affected side, and hemodynamic instability. The pneumothorax can also be seen on ultrasound or x-ray.

100. A: Patients with diseases that can affect their ability to properly breathe (because of muscle impairment) are at greater risk for respiratory acidosis because of the inadequate ventilation. Croup, bronchitis, and hypothyroidism do not cause paralysis of the respiratory muscles; however, Guillain-Barré can. When patients are insufficiently able to breathe, excessive amounts of carbon dioxide build up in the blood and the body produces excess H_2CO_3 in an attempt to compensate. This removes hydrogen from the blood, causing it to become more acidic.

101. C: Sellick maneuver involves applying pressure to the cricoid, using the thumb and forefinger, which is what was described, so this choice can be ruled out. This is to help close off the esophagus, preventing aspiration, in patients who have not been fasting (usually in emergency situations). Medications are administered to relax the smooth muscles and anesthetize the patient before intubation. Capnography can verify placement of the ETT, so if the physician is just now performing Sellick maneuver, the patient is not yet intubated.

102. B: CPAP is a great tool in patients who have congestive heart failure because the consistent positive pressure during respirations reduces both preload and afterload pressures on the heart. The effort required to breathe is also much lower, reducing the need for intubation and ventilation. BiPAP machines also provide positive pressure, but increases the pressure during the patient's inspiration. Tracheostomy may become necessary in the event that the patient destabilizes and is no longer able to ventilate on his/her own. LMA is not an appropriate method of ventilation in this situation.

103. D: The normal partial pressure for oxygen is greater than 80 mm Hg.

104. A: Ipratropium is an anticholinergic and common adverse effects are dry mouth, nose, and eyes, and difficulty urinating. Nosebleeds and nausea are also frequently reported by patients taking this class of drugs. The patient should be counseled, however, to report any visual changes, such as blurriness and halos.

105. B: An adolescent girl who is taking birth control pills and smokes has a much higher risk for developing deep venous thromboses. If untreated, a clot can break off and travel to the heart, lungs, and/or brain, and cause severe complications. In this case, her symptoms correlate with pulmonary embolus, a clot that has lodged in her lungs.

106. A: The patient's lowered pH indicates an acidotic condition, eliminating choices B and D. The elevated partial pressure of carbon dioxide in conjunction with the normal bicarbonate level indicates that this is a respiratory condition, not a metabolic one.

107. C: Given the injury to the ribs on the left side, be alert for potential injuries to the organs underneath. The liver and appendix are both on the right side of the body, but the spleen is on the left, tucked under the ribs. Injury to the small bowel is possible, but less likely to be a result of the rib injury because of the location of the bowel in relation to the ribs. Splenic rupture is the best choice here.

108. D: When applying a 12-lead ECG, 10 electrodes are placed around the body to measure the rhythm and rate of cardiac activity. One lead is placed on each of the 4 limbs, and 6 leads are placed around the heart, known as precordial leads. V1 is placed at the fourth intercostal space, on the right sternal border. V2 is placed also on the fourth intercostal space, but on the left sternal border. V4 is placed next, on the fifth intercostal space, midclavicularly. V3 is then placed midway between V4 and V2. V5 is next, horizontal to V4 but on the left anterior axillary line. V6 is placed on the midaxillary line along the same plane.

109. C: During an ECG, right-sided leads are placed at the mirror image location of their left counterparts. So, where a V6 lead is placed at the fifth intercostal on the left midaxillary line, a right-sided V6 lead is also on the fifth intercostal space but at the right midaxillary line.

Right-sided leads are used to look for ST elevations in suspected right ventricular infarctions.

110. A: Calculating MAP is simple: multiple the diastolic pressure by 2 and add the systolic pressure. Divide the sum by 3 to determine the MAP. In the question, the calculation would be as follows: $(64 \times 2 + 100)/3 = (128 + 100)/3 = 228/3 = 76$. A normal MAP is between 70 and 100 mm Hg. MAP is a measure of cardiac output and peripheral resistance. Cardiac output is heart rate and stroke volume.

111. A: The radial artery is the one most commonly used for arterial lines. However, before insertion, the Allen test (or a Doppler study) should be used to ensure adequate collateral circulation. Depress both the radial and ulnar arteries for a few moments until the hand blanches. Slowly release one of the arteries and observe the hand flushing as blood returns to the hand. Repeat, but this time, release the other artery and observe for the same flushing. If normal color and therefore blood flow return, this is a "positive" test. If color does not return the test is "negative" and there is not safe blood supply to the hand to use it. Radial is preferable to femoral lines when possible due to risk for infection.

112. A: Length-based resuscitation tape is sometimes necessary in emergency situations when an exact weight cannot be obtained on a child. The tape approximates the child's weight and dosage of commonly used emergency medicines based on height. The red end of the tape should be aligned with the top of the head and extended along the length of the child from head to heel, and follow readings accordingly. *Broselow* tape is a commonly used brand in which the different lengths are broken into easy to read, color-coded sections.

113. C: Elevating the patient's chest helps to stabilize the heart against the chest wall, and is the correct position for a patient about to undergo pericardiocentesis. Local anesthetic should be given, and the chest and epigastric areas prepped with povidone-iodine solution. Sometimes, insertion of an NG tube is necessary to relieve abdominal pressure and distension. The practitioner should monitor the ECG very closely to ensure that the ventricular wall is not punctured.

114. A: Aneurysms are classified according to where the weakness is located and how the vessel bulging presents. True aortic aneurysms involve all 3 layers of the aortic wall, while a false aneurysm is one that only affects the 2 outermost layers of the vessel wall. In a dissecting aneurysm, the vessel walls split, allowing blood to leak into and between the different layers. A fusiform aneurysm occurs when there is a weakness and bulging around the entire perimeter/circumference of the aorta.

115. D: Endotracheal administration of medication may be necessary in emergency situations in which venous access cannot be immediately established. The administered dose should be approximately twice what was ordered and may need to be mixed in diluent to increase effectiveness. AHA recommends a total volume of 10 mL for adults, 5 mL for children, and 1 mL for infants.

116. D: Patients with class III heart failure are symptomatic, even with mild exertion, and have significant restrictions in their activities in daily living as a result. Most patients with this class heart failure will be on an ACE inhibitor or beta blocker, a diuretic, and digoxin (if needed for contractility). This patient however, presents a medication list with two of the same class of ACE inhibitor. This should be investigated further, as it could be a medication

error, especially as the patient has multiple doctors prescribing medications. Insulin is often used in conjunction with metformin to manage diabetes.

117. B: Quinidine is a medication used for cardioversion from an atrial flutter rhythm to normal sinus rhythm. It is administered at a rate of up to 0.25 mg/kg/min IV, or 190 to 380 mg IM. Digoxin is not an antiarrhythmic and will not cardiovert a patient. Lidocaine is a ventricular antiarrhythmic and will therefore not correct an atrial dysrhythmia. Adenosine is typically used to convert supraventricular tachycardia (SVT) into sinus rhythm and is not usually effective on atrial flutter.

118. B: A patient who has had a myocardial infarction, or heart attack, will have many changes in his lab values and ECG. All 3 lab indicators of an MI, CK-MB, troponin, and myoglobin, will begin to rise within a few hours from the initial cardiac event and will peak at various times. Troponin and CK-MB levels will peak within about 24 hours, and myoglobin within 12 hours. Troponin will stay elevated for up to a few weeks after the initial event. There are other reasons why the levels of these enzymes would be increased, but you can rule an MI out if you do not see them rise.

119. A: To assess jugular venous pressure, the patient's head should be elevated and turned to the right. This allows the practitioner to directly observe the left jugular vein and its height. A patient with increased jugular pressure would have a height of 4 cm or greater, which indicates increased right atrial pressure or right-sided heart failure. When assessing the jugular veins, make sure to position the light appropriately so that you can see the vein and its shadows.

120. C: Indications for a thoracotomy in the ED include penetrating or blunt trauma to the abdominal or chest, nonresponsiveness to CPR in the nontrauma patient, and air embolism. An airway should be established and external chest compressions should continue until the first incision is made. After induction, the physician will make the first incision, usually in an anterolateral direction in the fourth intercostal space.

121. D: Simvastatin is a statin drug and is excreted by the liver. Patients should be advised of the potential for serious complications and instructed to look for symptoms of damage. Symptoms of liver damage include jaundice, or yellowing of the skin or eyes, abnormal bleeding, or severe fatigue. The other GI effects listed are not concerning unless they are severe or bothering the patient. The patient should also be aware of the possible need for regular blood testing to ensure that the liver is functioning well.

122. A: A patient with stable angina should be aware of his symptoms and do his best to lie down and relax. Decreased activity is usually beneficial in reducing the severity and occurrence of symptoms. Taking an aspirin or going to the ED is not necessary unless the patient's symptoms do not dissipate or they worsen with rest.

123. B: The only abnormal characteristic of the ECG strip is the rate of 42 bpm, which would classify the rhythm as a bradycardia. A rhythm with a regular P wave and QRS complex, and a 1:1 ratio of P waves to QRS complexes is characterized as a sinus, or regular rhythm. If the rate were between 60 and 100 bpm, the strip would be classified as a normal sinus rhythm. A patient in first-degree AV block would show similar characteristics on the ECG strip, except that the PR interval would be greater than 0.2 seconds. This type of arrhythmia is produced when conduction from AV node to ventricles is slower than normal.

124. A: Atrial flutter occurs when the atrium is pumping faster than the AV node is able to conduct the impulse to the ventricles. The rhythm is characterized by a saw-toothed P wave, because the atrial conduction is rapid and erratic. QRS waves would be normal because ventricular contraction is not affected by the abnormal atrial contractions. However, the ratio would be increased, because the rate and frequency of atrial contractions would be much higher than ventricular contraction. A patient in atrial fibrillation would display F waves and an unmeasurable P:QRS ratio.

125. D: Digoxin has a stronger and more potent effect in a patient who is dehydrated. Therefore, patients who are taking digoxin should take it with a large glass of water and make an effort to stay hydrated during the day. Drinking alcohol and caffeine in excess could be dangerous if the patient did not compensate and drink extra water. Becoming dehydrated is the correct answer.

126. D: This child has epiglottitis, a medical emergency. He appears anxious and agitated due to partial airway obstruction and air hunger. Children with epiglottitis appear quite ill and often have high fevers. They assume a tripod position with the chin jutting forward in an attempt to increase movement of air into the lungs. Difficulty swallowing causes pooling of saliva and drooling. This child was taken to the OR and a laryngoscopic exam under anesthesia revealed a swollen, red epiglottis. The physician then intubated the child. Although one should strive to intubate under controlled conditions in the OR, it may be necessary to intubate in the ED if the child's condition is deteriorating. One should not attempt to inspect the throat, do a strep test, give medication, or force the child to lie down because these maneuvers may trigger an airway spasm and lead to total airway occlusion. Racemic epinephrine is used for treatment of croup. Although inspiratory stridor may also occur with croup, when the other symptoms are taken into account, they are more diagnostic of epiglottitis.

127. C: Abdominal aortic aneurysms are most common in men within the 50 to 80 year range. When pain occurs, it is usually deep in character and mainly in the back. Aneurysms occur in people who have high blood pressure, especially if they are smokers. If rupture is imminent or if the aneurysm is expanding rapidly, it commonly causes pain. In addition, abdominal palpation reveals tenderness. An abdominal mass and a midline abdominal bruit are also common findings. The intraoperative risk of death is 50% when rupture has occurred. If repaired prior to rupture, a stent can be positioned inside the aneurysm by threading a catheter into the aorta via the femoral artery.

128 C: Early symptoms of Crohn's disease include chronic diarrhea (at times bloody), cramping abdominal pain, weight loss, fever, and anorexia. During flare-ups the patient may also have joint pain and inflammation. It commonly occurs between ages 15 to 25 years and can occur in any part of the digestive tract. However, it appears most often in the terminal ileum. Perianal fistulae are a common complication of Crohn's disease. While some of the symptoms of irritable bowel syndrome (IBS) may be similar, patients with IBS generally appear healthy and do not have systemic symptoms or fistula formation. Diverticulitis most often affects the sigmoid colon and occurs in people older than 40.

129. B: This patient is having a dystonic drug reaction. Drugs that most likely precipitate dystonic reactions include haloperidol, promethazine, chlorpromazine, and metoclopramide (which this patient was taking). An acute dystonia may be confused with a partial seizure or

- 49 -

psychotic posturing, but based on the dramatic response to diphenhydramine and the fact the patient is at risk while taking metoclopramide, it makes the diagnosis of dystonic reaction more likely. Transient ischemic attacks and dystonic reactions do not share any similarities.

130. A: A simple laceration of the frenulum of the upper lip is not serious and does not need to be repaired. It heals well on its own, does not require sutures or cauterization, and will not result in speech impairment. In addition, applying EMLA cream to an open wound is contraindicated. The objective is to rule out other injuries and to reassure the patient that the injury will heal spontaneously.

131. B: When measuring pulsus paradoxus, use the blood pressure cuff in the standard manner, but deflate the cuff more slowly than usual. Note the pressure at which the initial Korotkoff sounds are heard only during expiration. Continue slow deflation, and note the pressure where the Korotkoff sounds are initially heard throughout the respiratory cycle. A patient has a significant pulsus paradoxus if the difference between the two measurements is more than 10 mmHg.
Pulsus paradoxus is common in moderate to severe cardiac tamponade and several conditions such as pulmonary embolism, constrictive pericarditis, restrictive cardiomyopathy, and severe obstructive pulmonary disease. A patient with cardiac tamponade may not have pulsus paradoxus if he has elevated left ventricular pressure from a preexisting disease.

132. C: To elicit Murphy's sign, the examiner palpates the right costal area and tells the patient to take a deep breath. The gallbladder then descends onto the examiner's fingers, causing pain. When an inflamed gallbladder reaches the examiner's hand, the patient may suddenly cease inspiration. This is referred to as inspiratory arrest. Murphy's sign is also used to diagnose carcinoma of the gallbladder. Murphy's sign can also be shown sonographically. In this method, an ultrasound transducer is used to palpate the right subcostal area while the patient takes a deep breath. The transducer shows the gallbladder descending at the time of inspiratory arrest. Murphy's sign is not associated with any of the other answer choices.

133. D: A pertussis culture is performed by inoculating special media with a specimen of nasopharyngeal secretions collected with a calcium alginate swab or a Dacron swab. The specimen is incubated for 10 to 14 days. Cultures could be negative in the early stages of the disease due to the fastidious nature of the organism. Also note that a culture may be falsely negative if obtained after the fourth week of illness. A positive culture is diagnostic. Specimens collected in the manner described in the other answer choices would be invalid because they were not from the nasopharynx and were not collected properly.

134. B: When preparing to remove a tick, wear protective gloves. Grasp the tick with fine-tipped tweezers and slowly pull up with steady pressure until the mouth of the tick separates from the skin. After removing the tick, disinfect the attachment site and wash your hands. Using heat, cautery, or occlusive techniques is usually not effective and could increase the risk of infection.

135. D: A patient has hyperkalemia when the serum potassium is greater than 5.1. Mechanisms for the development of hyperkalemia include decreased excretion of potassium, shifting of intracellular potassium to the extracellular fluid, or excessive intake

of potassium. Cardiovascular effects include a decrease in blood pressure, bradycardia, and irregular heart rate. The effects on ECG are wide QRS complexes, flat P waves, peaked T waves, and long PR intervals.

136. A: During thyroid surgery, the parathyroid glands may be injured or accidentally removed because of their proximity to the thyroid. This results in hypocalcemia. Common findings of hypocalcemia include muscular twitches, cramps, and even tetany. Numbness can also occur in various areas, including the nose, lips, and extremities. It commonly causes anxiety and irritability. Although hypocalcemia is associated with a prolonged QT interval on ECG, long QT syndrome is a cardiac rhythm disorder causing tachycardia and disordered heartbeats, which are not seen in this patient. The clinical information provided in this patient's case does not definitively support a diagnosis of acute MI. Recurrent laryngeal nerve damage can occur as a result of thyroid surgery and cause a hoarse voice if nerve damage is unilateral or loss of voice and breathing difficulties if nerve damage is bilateral. This patient does not demonstrate these findings.

137. C: Brain hemorrhages or contusions frequently occur in multiple areas as a result of a single blow. This is known as an acceleration–deceleration mechanism of injury. If the initial blow occurs in the occipital area, this often also results in injury to the frontal or anterior temporal lobes. In this instance, a severe blow to the back of the patient's head injures the occipital area of the brain (coup injury), but also causes the brain to jar forward inside the skull, causing contusion to the frontal areas of the brain (contrecoup injury).

138. C: This clinical scenario describes a prolapsed umbilical cord. In these cases, the cord may be palpable or visible. Entrapment of the cord between the presenting part and the amnion or compression as the cord protrudes through the cervix compromises blood circulation. Prolapse results in a decrease in fetal circulation. The patient should be instructed *not* to push because this puts more pressure on the cord and further compromises fetal circulation. The maneuvers described in answers A, B, and D may help relieve pressure on the cord. Other interventions include monitoring the baby for hypoxia, applying digital pressure on the presenting part to decrease pressure on the cord, administering oxygen to the mother, and preparing for a Cesarean section.

139. A: Signs of bacterial vaginosis are a thin grayish-white vaginal discharge and a fishy odor. Bacterial vaginosis (BV) is the most prevalent form of vaginitis in sexually active women. The amine test (or whiff test) consists of adding 10% potassium hydroxide to a specimen of the vaginal discharge, resulting in a distinctive fishy odor. Another finding is the presence of clue cells (vaginal epithelial cells with ragged borders). The causative organism, *Gardnerella vaginalis* can be found in women who are not sexually active and who do not have BV. Culture is, therefore, not recommended. Trichomonas is associated with a larger amount of discharge that causes severe itching and is yellow, gray, or greenish and frothy.

140. A: A thick, foul-smelling unilateral nasal discharge is highly suggestive of a foreign body in the nose. Young children often place small objects inside a nostril unbeknownst to parents, who usually suspect an infection because of the bad odor. The discharge becomes foul smelling when the foreign body has been in the nose for a prolonged period. Although purulent drainage and nasal obstruction can be seen with a sinus infection, it is bilateral and associated with antecedent cold symptoms. In addition, sinusitis is not common at this age. An URTI is usually associated with other symptoms such as malaise, cough, sneezing,

headache, scratchy throat, and watery eyes. Allergies are associated with bilateral nasal symptoms, itchy/reddish eyes, and a previous history of similar symptoms that usually flare up seasonally.

141. D: Budesonide is an inhaled corticosteroid used in the maintenance treatment of asthma. Amiodarone treats ventricular fibrillation and unstable ventricular tachycardia. Lidocaine and verapamil are also antidysrhythmic drugs. Other categories of drugs used in cardiopulmonary resuscitation are calcium channel blockers, parasympatholytics such as atropine, sympathomimetic drugs such as epinephrine or isoproterenol, and alkalotic agents such as sodium bicarbonate.

142. A: A baby who is not old enough to walk is not likely to fracture a bone on his own. In this age group, a spiral leg fracture is suggestive of physical abuse. Spiral fractures occur when an abuser twists an extremity with a wringing motion. In older children and adults, a spiral fracture results from a twisting motion of the leg while the foot is firmly planted on the ground. Another clue to abuse is the presence of multiple old or new fractures on skeletal survey radiographs. A Galeazzi fracture occurs commonly in adults, resulting either from a fall or a blow to the lateral wrist and distal radius. A Monteggia fracture occurs on the proximal ulna and includes dislocation of the head of the radius.

143. C: Most nosebleeds originate from the anterior septum through irritation or erosion of the blood vessels in Kiesselbach's plexus. The key component to stopping the bleeding is to put pressure on the anterior septum by pinching the nostrils shut for at least 10 minutes. The patient should be instructed to breathe through the mouth during this time. Leaning the patient backward is a common mistake. This allows blood to flow into the throat and cause ingestion of blood, leading to gastrointestinal (GI) upset. Applying pressure to the bony part of the nose is not helpful, as that is not the site of the bleeding. Another common misconception is that ice will stop a nosebleed.

144. A: The correct placement of the precordial leads is as follows:
   V1 at the right sternal border in the fourth intercostal space
   V2 at the left sterna border in the fourth intercostal space
   V3 midway between V2 and V4
   V4 left midclavicular line in the fifth intercostal space
   V5 horizontal to V4 at the left anterior axillary line
   V6 horizontal to V5 at the left midaxillary line

145. B: Metformin is a drug that helps decrease blood sugar by lowering the amount of glucose produced by the liver. It also enhances utilizations of glucose at the cellular level and decreases the amount of glucose absorbed from food. Lactic acidosis is a very rare side effect of metformin, but when it occurs, it is fatal 50% of the time. Alcohol increases the risk of lactic acidosis while taking metformin. Other risk factors for developing lactic acidosis while on metformin include heart failure and impaired renal function.

146. D: Beta blockers decrease the heart rate. Beta blockers block beta 1 receptors (heart muscle) as well as beta 2 receptors (vascular and bronchial muscles). In addition to decreasing the heart rate, they cause a decrease in blood pressure and a decrease in cardiac output, both with exertion and at rest. These actions make beta blockers appropriate for treatment of hypertension, angina, and chronic cardiac failure. By causing blood vessel dilation, beta blockers *decrease* afterload. In this patient, a decrease in blood pressure

would be a desired effect of the beta blocker. Pulsus alternans is a pulse that regularly alternates between strong beats and weak beats without affecting the pulse rate, but is not a side effect of beta blockers. Impotence is a common side effect of beta blockers.

147. B: This patient has symptoms of morphine toxicity. In fact, she exhibits the "classic triad" of pupillary constriction, coma, and respiratory depression. After securing an airway and establishing venous access, the patient can be given IV naloxone, a narcotic antagonist. The patient may need repeated doses because of the short duration of action of naloxone. This is not an arrest situation because the patient has both pulse and respirations present.

148. C: Asthma should be treated acutely with a bronchodilator. An inhaled beta-2-receptor agonist, such as albuterol, would be appropriate. In more severe cases, an inhaled anticholinergic medication can also be used. Steroid inhalers and leukotriene inhibitors are used in maintenance/prophylactic therapy and, therefore, are not helpful in an acute situation. Nebulized therapy has several advantages, including quicker onset of action delivered directly to the lungs, fewer side effects, and easy administration. Diphenhydramine is not indicated for the treatment of asthma.

149. C: The usual incubation period for foodborne poisoning with ciguatoxin is about one to six hours. The infection is carried by fish (barracuda, grouper, snapper, and others). An affected person develops vomiting, diarrhea, and paresthesias after the ingestion of contaminated fish. The other answer choices presented are all associated with gastrointestinal manifestations, but they do not cause paresthesias. Botulism is also associated with neurologic findings, but those involve a descending paralysis.

150. D: The heart classically appears "water bottle"-shaped on x rays of patients with large pericardial effusions. When large enough, a pericardial effusion may cause cardiac tamponade and compromised heart function. A patient with pericarditis complains of pleuritic chest pain that dissipates by leaning forward. In general, pericarditis is mild and resolves with the aid of NSAIDs and corticosteroids. However, it can cause pericardial scarring and calcification, leading to constricted cardiac function.

151. C: The measurement of cardiac output is obtained by multiplying the heart rate by the stroke volume, and then divide by 1000. Cardiac output measurements are useful to evaluate ventricular function and effectiveness of pumping by the heart. It measures the quantity of blood pumped out of the ventricle per minute. Normal cardiac output ranges from four to eight liters per minute. In this case 50 ml/beat x 61 beat per minute = 3050 mL/minute. Divide this by 1000 as there are 1000mL in 1 L = 3.05, which is below normal.

152. D: Narcan is a short-acting narcotic antagonist that usually has to be given in repeat doses. It interferes with opiate receptors and thereby relieves respiratory depression and increases level of consciousness. Narcan can be given incrementally in doses of 0.2 mg until satisfactory improvement is seen. Routes of administration include IV, IM, SQ, or intranasally. In some cases, a continuous IV infusion is necessary.

153. C: The endotracheal (ET) tube size for a child can be calculated by taking the age in years and dividing by 4, and then adding 4 to that quantity. The equation is (age ÷ 4) + 4 = ET tube size. In this case, (4 ÷ 4) + 4 = 5. The ET tube size is 5.0.

154. C: A heparin overdose is treated with protamine. Vitamin K is the antidote for warfarin. Heparin overdose causes bleeding that can be life threatening. Petechiae and easy bruising are early signs of overdose. The condition progresses to overt bleeding such as epistaxis and hematuria. Heparin is administered by slow IV infusion at a maximum rate of 50 mg in a 10-minute period.

155. A: CSF protein is increased in patients with Guillain-Barré syndrome. This syndrome is thought to be an autoimmune condition that follows a viral or bacterial infection. Weakness begins in the lower extremities and ascends. If respiratory muscles are affected, the patient needs mechanical ventilation.

156. B: Melena is the medical term for black, tarry stools containing digested blood. It is a sign of upper-GI-tract bleeding, as seen in small bowel disease or peptic ulcers. Bleeding from the colon, rectum, and hemorrhoids is typically red.

157. B: A fracture of the cribriform plate of the ethmoid bone can cause a tear in the meninges with resultant leakage of CSF into the nose. Although a patient could have increased intracranial pressure in this scenario, it is not the direct cause of the CSF leak. Vasomotor rhinitis is associated with rhinorrhea in the absence of allergy or infection and is not associated with trauma.

158. A, C, and D: The aortic, tricuspid, and pulmonic areas are all locations where you can assess heart sounds. Purkinje fibers are not an area that can be ausculatated.

159. A, B, and C: The Broselow tape is a color-coded tape used to determine resuscitation drug dosages in infants and small children. The child is measured starting with the red end of the tape at the head and ending at the heel. The point where the heel touches the tape shows approximate weight, precalculated resuscitation drug doses, fluid doses, and equipment sizes.

160. C: The most common cause of hypoglycemia is an insulin reaction in diabetics. Tight blood sugar control puts a patient at risk for hypoglycemia. Answer choices A, B, and D are also associated with hypoglycemia, but they are not as common as C: Other less common causes include sepsis, tumors of the pancreas, and liver disease.

161. A: Femoral lines can be used to access central venous circulation in some patients. During cardiac arrest, a femoral line can be inserted without interfering with cardiac compressions. This makes it a good choice in an arrest situation. A femoral line is always assumed to be contaminated. An alternate site must be established after the patient is stable. Femoral line complications include infection and hematoma. They have a higher rate of infection than internal jugular lines and subclavian lines.

162. C: The Moro reflex is a normal action that is present at birth. It is typically triggered by an unexpected noise or touch and consists of outward flinging of both arms, followed by drawing the arms inward in an embracing posture. As the reflex ends, the action relaxes. Some babies let out a brief cry during the reflex. The Moro reflex disappears by four months of age. Many parents mistake this action for seizure activity. Infantile spasms are a type of seizure characterized by an abnormal electroencephalogram (EEG) pattern called hypsarrhythmia. These seizures consist of a sudden bending forward of the body and

- 54 -

stiffening of the extremities. Spasms may occur several hundred times a day. Cerebral palsy is a type of encephalopathy resulting from anoxic injury to the brain, often during delivery.

163. A: Pulmonary embolism (PE) occurs when one or more blood vessels in the lung are blocked by clots. Chest pain, dyspnea, hemoptysis, and syncope are all symptoms of pulmonary embolism. Other symptoms include wheezing, clammy skin, diaphoresis, weak pulse, and rapid heartbeat. Anticoagulant therapy is appropriate in the stable patient, however, it will not lyse an existing clot. It only prevents further clot propagation, and therefore allows the body to lyse its own clot naturally. INR goal is 2-2.5. The Joint Commission has stated that anticoagulants are more likely than other meds to cause harm due to complex dosing schedules, inefficient monitoring, and patient noncompliance.

164. A: Currant jelly stools are associated with an intussusception, a type of intestinal obstruction that results when one portion of the intestine "telescopes" into the adjacent section. About 80% of cases occur before age 24 months. Some patients may pass a stool containing mucus and blood, the so-called currant jelly stool. However, this finding is seen in only about 60% of infants; therefore, its absence does not rule out an intussusception.

165. D: The mortality rate for shaken baby syndrome (SBS) is closest to 50%. In SBS, an infant can have severe intracranial injury without external evidence of head trauma. Subdural hematomas and/or retinal hemorrhages in infants should raise suspicion of SBS. A nurse should be able to educate parents about the potentially fatal effects of shaking a baby. Some things you can emphasize are
    1. Never shake a baby up and down on your thigh, even playfully.
    2. Don't "play" with an infant by tossing him up in the air.
    3. Never shake an infant.

166. B: Battle's sign is indicative of a basilar skull fracture. It consists of ecchymosis over the mastoid area, usually manifested after 24 hours of injury. In addition to being ecchymotic, the area may also feel boggy. Other indicators of a basilar skull fracture are CSF otorrhea or CSF rhinorrhea.

167. D: A patient with an epidural hematoma has a torn middle meningeal artery. As the hematoma expands, it compresses the brain and leads to herniation and death unless treated immediately.

168. C: Be alert for entrapment of the extraocular muscles from a blowout fracture of the orbit. Blunt force to the face may cause fracture of the thin bone that forms the orbital floor and wall. Eye muscles could become trapped between broken bone fragments. It is important to assess for restricted or painful lateral or upward gaze. Some patients may also have crepitus at the site of fracture.

169. C: The pituitary gland is often called the master gland of the body because it influences the function of all endocrine glands. It has two sections, anterior and posterior. Oxytocin is produced by the posterior pituitary gland. The anterior pituitary produces ACTH, prolactin, and growth hormone. Other hormones produced by the anterior pituitary are follicle-stimulating hormone, thyroid-stimulating hormone, luteinizing hormone, and melanocyte-stimulating hormone. The posterior pituitary also produces vasopressin.

170. C: Patients in DKA need treatment for dehydration. Initial fluid replacement is usually accomplished with 0.9% saline by rapid infusion. When the blood glucose level comes down to the range of 250 to 300 mg/dL, 5% dextrose is added to the IV fluids. The life-threatening manifestations associated with DKA are dehydration, hyperglycemia (usually ranging from 300 to 800 mg/dL), acidosis, and electrolyte depletion.

171. D: Struvite stones are sometimes called "infection stones." These stones form in alkaline and ammonia-rich urine, and the urine is often alkaline and high in ammonia during a UTI. Cystine stones are quite rare and are seen in patients with genetic defects. Uric acid stones appear in patients who have gout. Calcium oxalate stones form when serum calcium levels are elevated or if there is an increase in calcium intake.

172. C: It is sometimes necessary to administer resuscitation drugs by the endotracheal route when IV access is inadequate. Epinephrine, atropine, naloxone, and lidocaine can all be given endotracheally. Calcium, sodium bicarbonate, and bretylium are not recommended for administration via endotracheal tube. There is a lack of pharmacokinetic data for these drugs.

173. C: SIDS is the sudden, unexpected death of an infant, usually while sleeping. Infants between two to four months of age are at highest risk. SIDS occurs less often after six months of age. Risk factors for SIDS include male gender, premature or low-birth-weight infants, siblings of SIDS infants, exposure to cigarette smoke, and sleeping on the stomach. Overheating may also play a role. Babies covered with several blankets or who sleep in overheated rooms are also at greater risk. Infants should be put to sleep on their backs, and parents should remove stuffed animals, pillows, bumper guards, and any other objects that could obstruct breathing.

174. D: In atrial fibrillation, both atria beat irregularly and out of sync with the ventricles. Rapid and irregular heart rate causes poor circulation to the body. Symptoms include palpitations, lightheadedness, weakness, chest pain, and shortness of breath. Thrombus formation is a complication because blood pools in the atria secondary to chaotic, irregular heartbeats. This, in turn, could lead to stroke. Atrial rates of 200 to 300 are not uncommon. Atrial fibrillation is treated with cardioversion followed by antiarrhythmic medications.

175. B: In a greenstick fracture, the break occurs only on one side of the shaft of a bone. This is common in children because their bones are flexible. When injured, the bone bends and cracks. Think of what happens when you attempt to break a green stick of wood. When you bend it, it cracks on one side, but it doesn't break all the way through.

Practice Test #2

Practice Questions

1. A client is a restrained passenger in a high-speed motor vehicle accident and is thought to have intra-abdominal bleeding. Which of the following is the best test to assess for hepatic or splenic rupture if the patient is relatively stable?
    a. Ultrasound
    b. CBC
    c. MRI
    d. CT

2. A six-week-old male infant is brought by his parents with a several day history of worsening projectile vomiting. What congenital abnormality should be considered?
    a. Toxic megacolon
    b. Appendicitis
    c. Pyloric stenosis
    d. Anal atresia

3. A client has an obstruction of the sphincter of Oddi from a gallstone. What is the most common complication of this condition?
    a. Appendicitis
    b. Pancreatitis
    c. Cholecystitis
    d. Hepatitis

4. A client with suspected appendicitis has pain in the right lower quadrant when palpated in the left lower quadrant. What is this diagnostic test called?
    a. Psoas sign
    b. Rovsing's sign
    c. Kernig's sign
    d. Brudzinski's sign

5. A client with an intestinal obstruction has a nasogastric tube placed in the ED. Which of the following acid-base disorders does this place the client at risk for?
    a. Respiratory acidosis
    b. Respiratory alkalosis
    c. Metabolic acidosis
    d. Metabolic alkalosis

6. A client has hypovolemia due to penetrating abdominal trauma. What is the best method for rapid fluid resuscitation?
    a. Large bore peripheral IV
    b. Femoral line central line
    c. Subclavian central line
    d. Jugular central line

7. An elderly client presents with profuse diarrhea for one week in a nursing home. She has recently recovered from an ICU stay the previous month for pneumonia and was on antibiotics for one month. Which of the following is the most likely organism for her diarrheal infection?
    a. Escherichia coli
    b. Clostridium difficile
    c. Staphylococcus aureus
    d. Staphylococcus pneumoniae

8. A client with abdominal pain has an upright KUB film that shows air under the diaphragm. Which of the following is the most likely cause?
    a. Intra-abdominal bleeding
    b. Bowel perforation
    c. Bowel obstruction
    d. Intussusception

9. Which of the following signs is NOT considered part of Charcot's triad of cholangitis?
    a. Fever
    b. Jaundice
    c. Elevated WBC
    d. RUQ tenderness

10. A client with chronic alcoholism presents with an acute upper GI bleed. What primary diagnosis should be considered?
    a. Esophageal varices
    b. Cholecystitis
    c. Pancreatitis
    d. Bowel perforation

11. Although Crohn's disease and ulcerative colitis can both cause inflammatory diseases of the colon, which other organ can be affected by Crohn's disease?
    a. Liver
    b. Spleen
    c. Stomach
    d. Lungs

12. An elderly client with LLQ pain, cramping in nature, is likely suffering from which of the following disorders?
    a. Appendicitis
    b. Meckel's diverticulum
    c. Hirschsprung's megacolon
    d. Diverticulitis

13. A client is having an ultrasound to evaluate for cholecystitis and has pain in the RUQ on expiration with the ultrasound probe in place. What is this sign called?
    a. Murphy's sign
    b. Psoas sign
    c. Rovsing's sign
    d. Battle sign

14. You are caring for a patient in the ED with heart failure exacerbation. The patient has dyspnea, fatigue and pulmonary edema. You know that the overall goal in treating heart failure is to:
   a. Improve the patient's cardiac function
   b. Assist the heart with remodeling
   c. Prevent further damage/exacerbations
   d. Increase intracardiac pressures

15. In addition to decreasing pain, morphine is given to patients with chest pain to improve which of the following hemodynamic parameters?
   a. Contractility
   b. Heart rate
   c. Preload
   d. Afterload

16. A patient is brought in by ambulance following an ATV wreck, during which he was thrown from the vehicle and hit a tree. Now, in the ED the patient's blood pressure has dropped significantly, he is complaining of difficulty breathing and his neck veins are obviously distended. On auscultation his heart sounds are muffled. The nurse knows these are signs of:
   a. Pericardial effusion
   b. Tension pneumothorax
   c. Pulmonary embolism
   d. Cardiac tamponade

17. A patient presents to the ED with chest pain. ECG shows ST elevation myocardial infarction. The patient is being prepped for the cardiac catheterization. What factors should decide if this patient will end up getting angioplasty, stents, or bypass surgery (choose all that may apply)?
   a. Patient presenting symptoms
   b. Physician preference
   c. Number of arteries blocked
   d. Degree of narrowing of arteries

18. What is the deciding factor as to whether a patient with a myocardial infarction is a candidate for thrombolytic therapy?
   a. Amount of ST elevation on EKG
   b. Severity of chest pain
   c. Troponin results
   d. CK/MB results

19. A patient presents to the ED with fatigue that he says has been getting worse for the last two weeks. On the cardiac monitor, the patient is noted to be in atrial fibrillation, with a ventricular rate of 140. Blood pressure is 146/86. The patient does not have any cardiac or medical history. What medication does the nurse expect to give in the ED in this scenario?
   a. ibutilide
   b. diltiazem
   c. warfarin
   d. digoxin

20. Which of the following patients does not have a contraindication to administration of thrombolytic therapy?
   a. 50-year-old client with an active GI bleed
   b. 45-year-old client who had a hip replacement one week previously
   c. 55-year-old client on chronic aspirin therapy
   d. 60-year-old client with a hemorrhagic stroke one month previously

21. In a client with blunt chest trauma from a high-speed motor vehicle accident, a finding of a widened mediastinum on chest x-ray should prompt the consideration of which of the following diagnoses?
   a. Flail chest
   b. Aortic dissection
   c. Pulmonary contusion
   d. Ruptured esophagus

22. A client has atrial flutter and is hemodynamically unstable. What is the most appropriate intervention?
   a. Cardioversion
   b. Lidocaine IV
   c. Bretylium IV
   d. Magnesium IV

23. A client with chest pain suddenly loses consciousness and shows ventricular fibrillation on the cardiac monitor. After calling for the code team, what is the next appropriate response?
   a. Intubation
   b. Lidocaine IV
   c. Epinephrine IV
   d. Defibrillation

24. A client with asystole has been intubated and had an IV placed. What is the first medication to be used in the code for this client?
   a. Bretylium
   b. Morphine
   c. Atropine
   d. Cardizem

25. A client with a stab wound to the chest is diagnosed with a pneumothorax. Which of the following is the treatment for this condition?
   a. Chest tube placement
   b. Endotracheal intubation
   c. Nasotracheal intubation
   d. Cricothyroidotomy

26. A patient with heart failure presents to the ED with pulmonary congestion, peripheral edema, and JVD. In treating this patient you will avoid which medication(s)?
   a. Digoxin
   b. NSAIDs
   c. Beta Blockers
   d. Opioids

27. What infectious heart condition is commonly seen in IV drug users?
    a. Pericarditis
    b. Cardiac tamponade
    c. Endocarditis
    d. Myocarditis

28. After intubating a client, aside from auscultation of the lung fields, what bedside technique can be used to assure placement of the endotracheal tube into the trachea and not the esophagus?
    a. Palpation
    b. CO2 monitoring of expiratory breath
    c. Pulse oximetry
    d. Pulmonary function testing

29. A client is in the ED after a blunt cardiac injury when the nurse notes a rhythm change and on investigation the nurse realizes the patient is having pulseless electrical activity (PEA). After CPR has been in progress for some time, without successful resuscitation the physician decides to do an emergency thoracotomy. Which of the following is untrue about this procedure?
    a. Closed chest compression should continue until the incision is made.
    b. Incision is usually anterolateral into the 4th intercostal space.
    c. Keep ventilating the patient during the opening of the pleura.
    d. Be prepare to remove clots from a hemothorax manually, with suction and towels.

30. An elderly client with a long history of insulin-dependent diabetes arrives at the ED with the complaint of dizziness for the previous week. EKG analysis shows her heart rate in the low 40's with transient episodes of increases up to 120. What is her likely diagnosis?
    a. Stroke
    b. Sick sinus syndrome
    c. Pericarditis
    d. Endocarditis

31. A 42-year-old woman is brought to the emergency department, with a sudden change in neurologic status. The patient's neurologic status, including the Glasgow Coma Scale, is quickly evaluated. Eye opening is to verbal stimuli. She is able to answer questions, but she is confused. She is able to follow commands weakly bilaterally. What is her score on the Glasgow Coma Scale?
    a. 11
    b. 12
    c. 13
    d. 14

32. You have the parents of a pediatric patient assist you to take the patient's temperature rectally. The patient's temperature is 100.0° F. The mom immediately begins to speak loudly stating "I knew my child had a fever and we just had to sit in the waiting room for over 2 hours!" After calmly listening to the mother, and addressing her concerns, what should you tell her about the temperature.What is the temperature considered a "fever" in pediatric patients when taken with a rectal thermometer?
   a. Temperature in infants is not considered a fever until it is over 101.2° F rectally.
   b. This is a fever, and you will get the physician right away.
   c. This is a fever, but it is not extremely elevated.
   d. Temperature in infants is not considered a fever until it is over 100.4° F rectally.

33. Which of the following would NOT be considered a major risk factor for coronary artery disease?
   a. Smoking
   b. Female sex
   c. Hypertension
   d. Diabetes

34. A 5-year-old client has a high fever, dysphagia, stridor, and sits leaning forward with the head extended. What potential infection should be considered?
   a. Appendicitis
   b. Sinusitis
   c. Epiglottitis
   d. Cholecystitis

35. A client arrives in the ED with status epilepticus. What is the most commonly used medication used to halt this seizure activity?
   a. lorazepam, one dose.
   b. lorazepam, every five minutes until seizures stop.
   c. temazepam
   d. librium

36. A first time seizure in a young adult born in Central America is likely due to which of the following conditions?
   a. Febrile seizure
   b. CVA
   c. Cysticercosis infection
   d. Aneurysm

37. A client is seen for anaphylactic shock. After the airway is secured, which of the following medications can be given subcutaneously to treat the condition?
   a. Atropine
   b. Corticosteroids
   c. Benadryl
   d. Epinephrine

38. You are caring for a patient who self administered her EpiPen. Which of the following indicates she needs more education regarding her EpiPen?
    a. "I wait until my symptoms of a reaction become severe before using my EpiPen, so that I am not using it unnecessarily."
    b. "I use my EpiPen, then call 911."
    c. "I inject my EpiPen into the muscle in my thigh."
    d. "I use my EpiPen when I feel tightness in my throat."

39. Which of the following findings on physical exam for a client with low back pain is most sensitive for the presence of a herniated disc?
    a. Tenderness of the spinal process at L5
    b. Tenderness of the posterior superior iliac spine
    c. Decreased range of motion
    d. Positive cross straight leg test

40. An elderly client presents to the ED with a red eye for 2 days. The pupil is dilated and unresponsive, and the intraocular pressure is over 50. What is the most likely cause?
    a. Acute glaucoma
    b. Conjunctivitis
    c. Iriditis
    d. Corneal foreign body

41. A patient presents in cardiogenic shock. The patient has a long history of heart failure, dysrhythmias, and valvular issues. The patient is in SVT with a heart rate of 200. No ST elevation noted on ECG. The patient is extremely dyspneic. Which of the following treatments would not be appropriate at this time?
    a. Mechanical ventilation
    b. Initiate hemodynamic monitoring
    c. Antidysrhythmics
    d. Thrombolytics

42. A 20-year-old client presents with complaints of severe neck pain and rigidity, fever, headache, and irritability. After the initial assessment, the nurse should prepare the patient for which of the following diagnostic tests?
    a. Blood culture
    b. Lumbar puncture
    c. Central line placement
    d. MRI of the head

43. Upon discharge from the ED, what is the best home assessment tool that an asthmatic client can use to gauge his/her lung functioning?
    a. Daily peak flow measurement
    b. Amount of cough
    c. Respiratory rate
    d. Fever

44. Which of the following medications is NOT to be used for treatment of acute asthma exacerbations?
   a. Solu-Medrol
   b. Singulair
   c. Albuterol
   d. Atrovent

45. A 20 year old patient taking Theophylline presents to the ER with irritability, restlessness, diarrhea, and tremors. She has been taking the medication for a few years and her blood work shows therapeutic levels. Which of the following would prompt the nurse to educate the patient further regarding using this medication?
   a. "I had to move my appointment back a day last time I was getting my theophylline level drawn because I had finals that day."
   b. "My ob-gyn said that if I decide to get pregnant we will probably consider trying another medication for my asthma. "
   c. "I just tried a Red Bull energy drink for the first time today, and it really helped me stay awake to study."
   d. "I also occasionally use a Levalbuterol (Xopenex) rescue inhaler."

46. A client presents with confusion, high potassium, and bradycardia. The patient is a 70kg average size male. Digoxin level is 1.6 ng/mL. What does this tell you?
   a. The patient has digoxin toxicity.
   b. The digoxin level is not therapeutic.
   c. The digoxin level is normal, search for another source for these symptoms.
   d. You do not have enough information to interpret the digoxin level.

47. A client is hit accidentally in the lateral chest with a golf club. He has an increased heart rate of 110 and a respiratory rate of 30. On exam he has decreased breath sounds on the left side. What is the most likely diagnosis?
   a. Myocardial contusion
   b. Pericardial tamponade
   c. Tension Pneumothorax
   d. Pulmonary embolism

48. Which of the four clients with pyelonephritis will likely need hospital admission for his/her treatment?
   a. A 25-year-old pregnant female
   b. A 40-year-old male with history of BPH
   c. A 75-year-old female with COPD
   d. A 65-year-old male with asthma

49. An elderly client is to be discharged from the ED with a diagnosis of abdominal pain due to constipation. Which of the following would NOT be a discharge recommendation?
   a. Increased exercise
   b. Increased fiber intake
   c. OTC stimulant laxatives daily
   d. Increased water intake

50. Which of the following medications for tachycardia can cause a brief episode of asystole after IV administration?
    a. Atropine
    b. Adenosine
    c. Lidocaine
    d. Verapamil

51. An elderly client arrives in the ED with confusion, fever, hypoxemia, elevated plasma lactate, acute renal failure, hypotension, and thrombocytopenia. Which of the following does this describe?
    a. Sepsis
    b. Severe Sepsis
    c. Septic Shock
    d. Multi-organ dysfunction syndrome

52. A pediatric patient is discharged with the diagnosis of chicken pox (varicella virus). Which of the following family members can the child to have contact with while infective?
    a. His uncle with symptomatic AIDS
    b. His grandfather on chemotherapy for colon cancer
    c. His pregnant sister
    d. His brother who has been immunized with the vaccine

53. Health care workers in the ED should be immunized with all of the following vaccines EXCEPT:
    a. Hepatitis A
    b. Hepatitis B
    c. Hepatitis C
    d. Influenza

54. An elderly client has a diagnosis of dementia. A nurse assesses the client using the Mini-Mental Status Exam. What score on this test is consistent with severe dementia?
    a. 25
    b. 13
    c. 29
    d. 30

55. A client has a contusion to the temporal area from an assault with a glass bottle. He complains of numbness in the side of his mouth and tongue. Which cranial nerve has been damaged?
    a. I
    b. III
    c. II
    d. V

56. Following penetrating trauma to the face, a client's right eye deviates inward and cannot move laterally. Which eye muscle has been damaged?
    a. Medial rectus
    b. Lateral rectus
    c. Inferior oblique
    d. Superior oblique

- 65 -

57. A client arrives in the ED having given birth in the ambulance. The mother and infant have stable vital signs, but the infant has signs of Erb's palsy with a flexed hand, palm facing backward, and a limp arm. Which neurological area was damaged during the delivery?
    a. Lower brachial plexus
    b. Upper brachial plexus
    c. Cerebellum
    d. Medulla oblongata

58. A client is to be discharged from the ED with a diagnosis of UTI. Which of the following would be considered an acceptable recommendation in treating this condition?
    a. One liter per day fluid restriction
    b. Ad lid carbonated soda
    c. Voiding every 8 hours
    d. OTC cranberry extract pills

59. Four clients are seen in the ED for fractures. Which of the following clients will likely need surgical intervention for the fracture?
    a. 7-year-old with femoral head fracture
    b. 40-year-old with 5th toe distal phalanx fracture
    c. 25-year-old with index finger tuft chip fracture
    d. 30-year-old with chip fracture of base of the 5th metatarsal head

60. A client on chronic kidney dialysis has missed 3 dialysis treatments due to social issues. What physical finding should be assessed to evaluate for hypervolemia?
    a. cardiac arrhythmias due to high potassium levels
    b. worsening of anemia and bone disease
    c. pedal edema and shortness of breath
    d. cramping and low blood pressure

61. A client with asthma and a respiratory rate of 30 is seen in the ED. For which acid-base disorder does this high respiratory rate place him at risk?
    a. Metabolic acidosis
    b. Metabolic alkalosis
    c. Respiratory acidosis
    d. Respiratory alkalosis

62. A patient with asthma and respiratory collapse is intubated in the ED. What is the next step in patient care?
    a. ABGs
    b. IVF bolus
    c. Pulmonary function testing
    d. Chest x-ray for endotracheal tube placement

63. An elderly client has a closed head injury from a fall. The patient's primary problem is that there is swelling. Swelling of the brain after a head injury is related to all of the following except:
    a. Interferes with perfusion.
    b. Causes hypoxia and hypercapnia.
    c. Triggers decreased blood flow.
    d. Increases intracranial pressure.

64. A client is seen in the ED with an overdose of acetaminophen (Tylenol). She is to be treated with acetylcysteine (Mucomyst). What is the appropriate administration route for Mucomyst?

    a. PO

    b. IV

    c. SQ

    d. PR

65. A client incurs a penetrating stab wound to the ventral forearm. The knife went all the way through the forearm and out the other side. The client's vital signs are stable and much of the bleeding has stopped. Which of the following diagnostic tests should be done to assess for damage to major arteries in the forearm?

    a. Ultrasound

    b. CT

    c. MRI

    d. Arteriogram

66. A 20-year-old male client has an acute onset of right-sided testicular pain and is suspected of having a testicular torsion. Which of the following tests should be used to assess the testicle?

    a. CT

    b. MRI

    c. Ultrasound

    d. Arteriogram

67. A pregnant client falls down a 20-foot flight of stairs. She is at 36 weeks gestation. What test can be done to assess for transmission of fetal blood cells into the maternal blood stream?

    a. Fetal heart tones

    b. Fetal autosomal aneuploidies

    c. Rhesus typing

    d. Kleihauer-Betke test

68. A female client who delivered her child 2 days previously and left the hospital the day before returns to the ED with the complaint of a severe posterior bilateral headache. She had an epidural for the delivery and has not been using any narcotic pain medications since she left the hospital. She does not have a fever and has a normal white blood cell count. What is the likely cause of her headache?

    a. Bacterial meningitis

    b. Spinal headache from CSF leak

    c. Viral meningitis

    d. Migraine headache

69. A client is having an MRI for evaluation of a possible cervical disc herniation. What should the nurse do before taking the client to the radiology department?

    a. Insert a large bore IV

    b. Shave posterior cervical area

    c. Inquire about contrast dye or iodine allergies

    d. Inquire about prior surgery.

70. A client with suspected sepsis needs blood cultures taken before initiation of antibiotic treatment. What is the best site for obtaining blood cultures?
    a. Femoral
    b. Antecubital fossa
    c. Popliteal fossa
    d. Wrist

71. A twenty-year-old male client has a minimally displaced clavicular midshaft fracture from a fall. Which of the following is the most appropriate treatment for this kind of fracture?
    a. Open reduction and internal fixation
    b. Surgical pinning
    c. Arm sling or figure-of-eight sling
    d. Casting

72. While performing a venipuncture, a nurse gets an accidental needle stick with a used needle. What is the next course of action for the nurse?
    a. As the risk of conversion of so small, the nurse need do nothing
    b Ask the patient if he has HIV
    c. Ask the patient if he has Hepatitis C
    d. Inform the ER supervisor

73. A client is seen in the ED after a sexual assault. Which of the following is NOT a recommendation for prophylactic therapy afterwards?
    a. Herpes virus treatment
    b. Emergency contraception
    c. HIV post-exposure prophylaxis
    d. Gonorrhea/Chlamydia treatment

74. A male client is seen in the ED for new onset of chest pain. Before a nitrate drip is started, which medication should the client be asked about using recently?
    a. Aspirin
    b. Hydrocodone (Vicodin)
    c. Sildenafil (Viagra)
    d. Coumadin

75. A celebrity client is in the ED after a motor vehicle accident. A nurse notices a medical assistant not involved in the patient's care trying to take pictures of the client on her cell phone. What should the nurse do next?
    a. Notify the ED supervisor of the HIPAA violation
    b. Ask the MA to stop
    c. Take the cell phone away from the MA
    d. Move the client to a remote room

76. An elderly client has sustained rib fractures of three adjacent ribs, both anteriorly and posteriorly. What intervention is not appropriate?
    a. Analgesia for pain relief
    b. Incentive spirometer
    c. Wrap the chest with tape
    d. Thoracotomy, if underlying injuries

77. Following exposure to a client with infectious TB, ED employees are given the Mantoux (PPD) skin test. How long after administration of the test should results be read?
    a. 6 to 12 hours
    b. 12 to 36 hours
    c. 48 to 72 hours
    d. 72 to 96 hours

78. A client with a pleural effusion needs both draining of the fluid and laboratory evaluation of the fluid. What procedure can be done for this condition?
    a. Thoracentesis
    b. Pericardiocentesis
    c. Lumbar puncture
    d. Peritoneal lavage

79. An elderly client has a skin tear on the forearm. What is the best dressing choice for this kind of skin trauma?
    a. Wet to dry dressing
    b. Vaseline gauze
    c. No dressing at all
    d. Tegaderm dressing

80. A female client is discharged with the diagnosis of anemia due to dysfunctional uterine bleeding. Which of the following is NOT a good source of iron for her diet?
    a. Potatoes
    b. Chicken
    c. Spinach
    d. Lamb

81. A family is brought into the ED after rescue from a structure fire. Which of the following clients should be monitored the closest for respiratory compromise?
    a. 20-year-old with a hoarse voice and soot around nostril
    b. 4-year-old with a burn on the palm of the hand
    c. 70-year-old with a burn to the chest and arm
    d. 6-month-old with an active cry

82. A 40-year-old female presents to the ED with pain and swelling in the right calf for one day. Which of the following would NOT be considered a high risk factor for deep vein thrombosis (DVT)?
    a. One pack per day smoking habit
    b. Diabetes
    c. Oral contraceptive use
    d. Recent immobilization of the limb due to a fracture

83. A male client in the ED states, "Jesus told me to come here." The client is likely suffering from which component of psychosis?
    a. Auditory hallucination
    b. Visual hallucination
    c. Flight of ideas
    d. Grandiosity

84. Which of the following children has a fracture likely caused by abuse?
    a. 8-year-old with Colles' fracture
    b. 3-month-old with spiral fracture of the femur
    c. 9-year-old with a clavicle fracture
    d. 18-year-old with avulsion fracture of ankle

85. A client with bipolar disorder is in a manic state and while interviewed skips from one topic to the next quickly with no apparent connection. Which of the following is this aspect of manic behavior?
    a. Echolalia
    b. Aphasia
    c. Poverty of speech
    d. Flight of ideas

86. Which of the following conditions would most likely cause high levels of anxiety in an ED client?
    a. Appendicitis
    b. Cholecystitis
    c. COPD exacerbation
    d. Finger fracture

87. A client is to be discharged from the ED after a panic attack. Which of the following medications would be most likely to have an immediate impact in controlling his symptoms?
    a. Bupropion (Wellbutrin)
    b. Paroxetine (Paxil)
    c. Lorazepam (Ativan)
    d. Fluoxetine (Prozac)

88. After an evaluation for a minor fall, a client tells the ED discharge nurse that he is homeless and has nowhere to go. What is her next appropriate course of action?
    a. Immediate discharge, as it is not the problem of the ED
    b. Psychiatry consult
    c. Social worker consult
    d. Have an orderly escort the client to a soup kitchen

89. A client is being treated for diabetic ketoacidosis. In addition to the insulin drip, what electrolyte should be added to the IV fluids?
    a. Magnesium
    b. Potassium
    c. Calcium
    d. Selenium

90. In which patient would you find a serum creatinine of 1.4 mg/dL probably normal for that patient?
    a. A young athletic male
    b. A 70 year old woman
    c. A cachectic AIDS patient
    d. A 45 year old male

91. The Allen test is used to detect blood supply in which part of the body?
    a. Foot
    b. Hand
    c. Neck
    d. Pelvis

92. A male client is brought to the ED by his wife. The man fell off a ladder 12 hours prior and sustained a closed head injury. He initially was without symptoms, but now 12 hours later has developed somnolence and weakness. What is the likely cause of his symptoms?
    a. Cranial fracture
    b. Epidural hematoma
    c. Semicircular canal disruption
    d. Subdural hematoma

93. An elderly client presents with a CVA and new onset right-sided weakness and aphasia. Which part of his brain has been compromised by the stroke?
    a. Right side of the cerebrum
    b. Left side of the cerebrum
    c. Cerebellum
    d. Medulla oblongata

94. Which of the following groups has the highest success rate for suicide attempts?
    a. Adult males
    b. Adult females
    c. Adolescent males
    d. Adolescent females

95. A client is brought to the ED with an intentional overdose. Which of the following medications requires close monitoring due to cardiac abnormalities?
    a. Acetaminophen (Tylenol)
    b. Ibuprofen (Motrin)
    c. Naprosyn (Aleve)
    d. Amitriptyline (Elavil)

96. A client with septic shock is treated in the ED. In addition to IV fluids, antibiotics, and airway support, which of the following is the vasopressor of choice for septic shock?
    a. dopamine (Intropin)
    b. epinephrine (Adrenaline)
    c. dobutamine (Dobutrex)
    d. norepinephrine (Levophed)

97. Due to increased risk of stroke, which of the following medications is NOT recommended for the use in treating hypertensive urgencies in the ED?
    a. Esmolol (Brevibloc)
    b. Labetalol (Normodyne)
    c. Diltiazem (Cardizem)
    d. Nifedipine (Procardia)

98. Asplenic clients should be immunized with which of the following vaccines to protect them against encapsulated bacteria?
    a. Influenza
    b. Pneumococcal
    c. MMR
    d. Varicella

99. A teenage client with fatigue and fever has been diagnosed with infectious mononucleosis. What should he be counseled to avoid while convalescing?
    a. Caffeine
    b. Contact sports
    c. Dental surgery
    d. Aspirin

100. A pregnant client presents with a headache. In addition to the blood pressure, what lab findings would be suggestive of pre-eclampsia?
    a. Tachycardia
    b. Hyponatremia
    c. Proteinuria
    d. Hematuria

101. A client presents to the ED with hematochezia. He is on warfarin (Coumadin) for a mechanical heart valve. Which of the following INR levels would indicate he is receiving a therapeutic dosage?
    a. 0.0 to 0.5
    b. 0.5 to 1.5
    c. 2.5 to 3.5
    d. 3.5 to 4.5

102. A client in the ED is being evaluated for iron deficiency anemia. This commonly results in a "microcytic" anemia with small red blood cells. What part of the CBC measures red blood cell size?
    a. Reticulocyte count
    b. Mean corpuscular volume
    c. Hemoglobin
    d. Hematocrit

103. A four-year-old client is undergoing resuscitation for hemorrhagic shock. What is the best site for infusion of fluids if a peripheral IV cannot be performed?
    a. Internal jugular central line
    b. Subclavian central line
    c. Femoral central line
    d. Interosseous line

104. A client with new-onset renal failure is found to have a critically high potassium value. Until hemodialysis can be arranged, which medication can be used to temporarily decrease the potassium level?
　　a. Furosemide (Lasix)
　　b. Sodium polystyrene sulfonate (Kayexalate)
　　c. Hydrochlorothiazide (HCTZ)
　　d. Amiodarone (Pacerone)

105. A pediatric client is diagnosed with streptococcal pharyngitis. The client has a history of anaphylactic allergy with penicillin. What would be the best choice for antibiotic treatment for this client?
　　a. Azithromycin (Z-Pak)
　　b. Nafcillin (Nallpen)
　　c. Amoxicillin (Amoxil)
　　d. Ciprofloxacin (Cipro)

106. A client in the ED complains of new-onset crushing chest pain. What EKG finding will make the decision to administer a thrombolytic difficult?
　　a. Supraventricular tachycardia
　　b. First degree AV block
　　c. Bradycardia
　　d. Left bundle branch block (LBBB)

107. A client with schizophrenia has uncontrolled movements of the tongue and lips (tardive dyskinesia). Long-term use of which of the following medications leads to this condition?
　　a. Paroxetine (Paxil)
　　b. Haloperidol (Haldol)
　　c. Lithium (Lithobid)
　　d. Valproic acid (Depakote)

108. After trauma in children, SCIWORA syndrome involves abnormalities not initially seen on x-ray in which part of the body?
　　a. Pelvis
　　b. Shoulder
　　c. Cervical spine
　　d. Hand

109. A client is seen in the ED for an overdose of lorazepam (Ativan). In addition to airway management and supportive measures, which of the following medications can be used to reverse the effects of this drug?
　　a. Naloxone (Narcan)
　　b. Acetylcysteine (Mucomyst)
　　c. Activated charcoal
　　d. Flumazenil (Romazicon)

110. A client is seen in the ED for an overdose of antifreeze (ethylene glycol). Which of the following medications can be used as a competitive inhibitor for the pathway of ethylene glycol?
    a. Naloxone (Narcan)
    b. Ethanol
    c. Activated charcoal
    d. Flumazenil (Romazicon)

111. Warfarin (Coumadin) is used as an anticoagulant for numerous conditions, including atrial fibrillation. If a client presents with overdose of Coumadin, which of the following can be given to the client to rapidly reverse the over anti-coagulation?
    a. Iron tablets
    b. Vitamin K
    c. Fresh frozen plasma (FFP)
    d. Platelets

112. A twenty-year-old client presents to the ED with chest pain. What part of the history would suggest a high possibility of coronary event?
    a. Recent cocaine use
    b. History of ASD as a child
    c. History of rheumatic fever as a child
    d. Recent antibiotic use

113. A client with pain at the base of the thumb is diagnosed with Dequervain's tenosynovitis. When he adducts his wrist with his thumb inside a clenched fist, he has pain. What is this diagnostic sign called?
    a. Tinel's sign
    b. Phalen's sign
    c. Finkelstein's test
    d. Allen's test

114. A teenage female client with a history of severe anxiety and psychiatric issues presents in the ED. On exam, she is noted to have numerous bald spots on her scalp and admits to intentionally pulling out her own hair. What is this psychiatric condition called?
    a. Anorexia nervosa
    b. Trichotillomania
    c. Kuru
    d. Bulimia

115. A client presents with a "tearing" chest pain and is suspected of having a thoracic aneurysm. What inherited connective tissue disease is associated with a higher risk of aortic aneurysms?
    a. Marfan's syndrome
    b. Trisomy 21
    c. Trisomy 18
    d. Sarcoidosis

116. A client is evaluated in the ED for new onset blindness due to a CVA. Which part of the brain has likely been affected?
    a. Anterior cerebrum
    b. Posterior cerebrum
    c. Cerebellum
    d. Medulla oblongata

117. A homeless client is found inebriated, supine, and with vomitus on his clothes by EMS. He is brought into the ED. If the patient has a patent airway, what is the most important next concern?
    a. Assessing cardiac rhythm and treating as needed
    b. Assessing adequacy of ventilations and treating as needed
    c. Assessing social status and referring for help
    d. Assessing gastrointestinal status due to vomitus

118. A client is seen for an acutely painful calf after a track meet. He felt a "pop" and cannot weight bear on the leg. Structural integrity of the calf can be assessed by squeezing the calf to determine if there is movement of the foot. What is this test called?
    a. Tinel's sign
    b. Thompson test
    c. Phalen's sign
    d. Rovsing's test

119. In adult clients with clean wounds, what time interval is recommended for tetanus boosters?
    a. 2 years
    b. 4 years
    c. 6 years
    d. 10 years

120. CPR is in progress on a patient in the ED. The patient has been receiving chest compressions and ventilations. Epinephrine 1 mg IV has been given 1 minute ago and now a biphasic defibrillator is connected to the patient showing ventricular fibrillation. What should be done next ?
    a. At the appropriate time in the cardiac cycle, give one shock at 150 J.
    b. Give one shock now at 150 J.
    c. At the appropriate time in the cardiac cycle, give one shock at 300 J.
    d. Give one shock now at 300 J.

121. A 10-year-old client has a second-degree burn to 1% of his body surface area. Which of the following body sites for burns of that magnitude would be LEAST likely to need early intervention by a plastic surgeon?
    a. Genitals
    b. Dorsal thigh
    c. Face
    d. Ventral hand

122. Following a severe auto-train accident, four clients are brought to the ED. Who among the following should be triaged for first treatment?
    a. 30-year-old client with respiratory distress and an open chest wound
    b. 60-year-old client with a severe open head wound and no pulse
    c. 45-year-old with a broken femur
    d. 5-year-old with a broken arm

123. A client has acute severe flank pain and is thought to have a kidney stone. What is the best diagnostic test for evaluation of this condition?
    a. Chest x-ray
    b. MRI
    c. Intravenous pyelogram (IVP)
    d. Intravenous discogram

124. A client with sickle cell disease is seen in the ED for a sickle cell crisis. Which of the following would not be considered routine first line treatment for a crisis?
    a. Oxygen
    b. Vitamin K
    c. IV hydration
    d. Pain medication

125. A client with a history of metastatic lung cancer presents to the ED with new- onset cough, chest pain, and dilated head and arm veins. What is the likely oncologic emergency?
    a. Spinal cord compression
    b. Superior vena cava syndrome
    c. Hypercalcemia
    d. Pericardial effusion

126. An elderly patient is brought into the ED with severe dehydration and confusion. You are have assessed him, drawn labs, and placed him on a cardiac monitor. You notice peaked T-waves on the monitor. No labs results are back yet when the patient starts having ventricular arrhythmias. You expect the physician to order:
    a. a bedside calcium level, and IV calcitonin if elevated
    b. a bedside sodium level, NS at 100 mL/hr
    c. a bedside potassium level, calcium gluconate IV if elevated
    d. a bedside glucose, and dextrose IV if low

127. Inappropriate production of which of the following hormones can lead to tachycardia and weight loss?
    a. Testosterone
    b. Estrogen
    c. Progesterone
    d. Thyroid hormone

128. In pediatric clients, cellulitis of which of the following body parts requires aggressive IV antibiotic therapy to avoid serious complications?
    a. Elbow
    b. Knee
    c. Orbits
    d. Auricle

129. A patient presents to the ED with pain in the arm. On x-ray it is discovered that there is a fracture. The patient states he does not recall any type of fall or event that should have led to this. Labs show decreased RBCs, decreased neutrophils, and decreased platelets. The patient complains of severe fatigue for more than two months. The nurse suspects:
    a. HIV/AIDS
    b. DIC
    c. Leukemia
    d. Non-hodgkins lymphoma

130. A client presents to the ED with a possible attempted suicide. The patient was found to have ingested multiple OTC medications including 4 Tylenol PM, an almost full bottle of aspirin, and a bottle of liquid pepto bismol. Treatment will include all of the following except:
    a. Sodium bicarbonate 2 mEq/kg.
    b. Electrolyte monitoring hourly.
    c. Whole bowel irrigation with sustained released tablets.
    d. acetylcysteine

131. A client is seen in the ED with a diagnosis of food poisoning. What is the most important ED action for this patient?
    a. Identification of tainted food
    b. Identification of causative bacteria organism
    c. Assessment of degree of dehydration
    d. Initiation of broad spectrum antibiotics

132. A client is seen in the ED for a severe laceration involving heavily contaminated debris. He is an immigrant from Africa and has never been immunized against tetanus. In addition to the tetanus toxoid vaccine, what else should he be given?
    a. Human tetanus immunoglobulin
    b. MMR vaccine
    c. Oral polio vaccine
    d. An extra tetanus vaccine dose

133. The Gardasil vaccine can be given to female teenage clients to prevent cervical cancer from which of the following causative organisms?
    a. Neisseria gonorrhea
    b. Chlamydia trachomatis
    c. HIV
    d. Human papilloma virus

134. An ED client has been diagnosed with gonorrhea. For which common concomitant infection should the client also be treated?
    a. Syphilis
    b. HIV
    c. Chlamydia
    d. Chancroid

135. An ED client is seen with a tick bite. It developed a small red papule that progressed to a bright red rash with a clear section in the middle. The client has also had a headache, fever and malaise. What is his likely diagnosis?
a. Babesiosis
b. Lyme disease
c. Rocky Mountain Spotted Fever
d. Cysticercosis

136. A client presents with a herpes zoster rash. In what part of the body can this cause potentially dangerous complications if not treated acutely?
a. Face
b. Trunk
c. Hand
d. Foot

137. A client is seen in the ED after a high voltage electrical injury. What is the most common cause of death due to electrical injuries?
a. Renal failure
b. Cardiac arrhythmias
c. Seizures
d. Burns

138. Prolonged Q-T intervals and a J-wave (Osborn wave) can occur in which of the following traumatic conditions?
a. Hyperthermia
b. Hypothermia
c. Drowning
d. Electrical injury

139. A client is seen who has acute mountain sickness due to rapidly ascending a mountain. In addition to supportive measures and oxygen, which of the following medications can be used to alleviate the condition?
a. Esmolol (Brevibloc)
b. Nitroglycerin (Tridil)
c. Aspirin
d. Acetazolamide (Diamox)

140. A child is seen with a barking cough and a fever and is diagnosed with croup. What is the most common causative organism?
a. Parainfluenza virus
b. Streptococcus
c. MRSA
d. Tetanus (Clostridium tetani)

141. What is the most common cause of painless lower GI bleeding in a young child?
a. Hirschsprung's megacolon
b. Anal atresia
c. Meckel's diverticulum
d. Pyloric stenosis

142. A pediatric client is seen with a "slapped cheek" rash and a fever and is diagnosed with erythema infectiosum. His family has been advised to keep the child away from pregnant women. Which is the causative organism for this condition?
   a. Parvovirus B19
   b. Streptococcus
   c. MRSA
   d. Measles virus

143. A 14 year old patient presents with weakness, headaches, fever, enlarged lymph nodes, enlarged spleen, and a persistent sore throat for three weeks. The physician orders an antibody test to check for:
   a. Strep throat
   b. Infectious mononucleosis
   c. Measles
   d. Mumps

144. A pediatric client is seen with a high fever, conjunctivitis, mouth lesions and a rash. He is diagnosed with Kawasaki's syndrome. What is the most serious potential complication of this disease?
   a. Hepatitis
   b. Renal failure
   c. Intestinal blockage
   d. Coronary artery disease

145. A pediatric client is seen with an acute encephalopathy. The patient has just gotten over chickenpox and now presented with vomiting, lethargy, spasms, and seizures. The mother tells you that during his illness he had high fevers that she treated with multiple over the counter medications. You suspect:
   a. Epidural hemorrhage
   b. Subdural hematoma
   c. Reye syndrome
   d. Child abuse

146. A client is seen during a trauma code. The physician states that he cannot get a peripheral IV and will try to perform a venous cutdown. Which site will likely be used for the cutdown?
   a. Ankle
   b. Knee
   c. Groin
   d. Neck

147. A client has a suspected Le Fort fracture after a serious motor vehicle accident. Which intervention is most important?
   a. CT scan of the face
   b. Assisting the physician to safely examine the face, neck, throat, and nares.
   c. Disimpact displaced fragments manually.
   d. Referral to surgeon for fixation.

148. A client who uses a jackhammer at work and has progressive numbness and tingling in the volar side of index and middle fingers is diagnosed with carpal tunnel syndrome. Which nerve is affected in this case?
 a. Radial
 b. Median
 c. Ulnar
 d. Sciatic

149. Following a fall, a client has pain and tenderness in the anatomical snuffbox of the wrist. Which is the most likely fractured carpal bone?
 a. Scaphoid
 b. Lunate
 c. Triquetrum
 d. Pisiform

150. A female client of childbearing age is seen in the ED for LLQ pain. Which of the following diagnoses is potentially life threatening if NOT diagnosed and treated promptly?
 a. Pyelonephritis
 b. Diverticulitis
 c. UTI
 d. Ectopic pregnancy

151. A 14-month-old client is seen in the ED with a "red jelly" stool and abdominal pain. The physician suspects that the client has intussusception. Which of the following is the best diagnostic test for this condition?
 a. CT
 b. MRI
 c. Barium enema
 d. Colonoscopy

152. An adult client is seen in the ED with abdominal pain, vomiting, and a high amylase level. He is diagnosed with pancreatitis. Which of the following is NOT a common cause for acute pancreatitis?
 a. Alcohol abuse
 b. Gallstones
 c. Hypertriglyceridemia
 d. Parainfluenza virus

153. A 50-year-old male client with a long history of alcohol abuse is seen in the ED for a fall. While there, he begins to exhibit symptoms of delirium tremens. Which of the following is the most appropriate medication for amelioration of these symptoms?
 a. Lorazepam (Ativan)
 b. Lithium (Eskalith)
 c. Thiamine IV
 d. Dietary supplementation

154. A client is seen after a severe motor vehicle accident. Due to trauma from the seat belt, he is felt to have a ruptured spleen. Which of the following signs is indicated by pain referred to the left shoulder due to left diaphragmatic irritation from a bleeding spleen?
  a. Tinel's sign
  b. Kehr's sign
  c. Phalen's sign
  d. Grey Turner's sign

155. A client falls off a ladder and lands on his heels, sustaining a calcaneal fracture. Given his mechanism of injury, which other body part should be closely assessed for impairment?
  a. Pelvis
  b. Lumbar spine
  c. Head
  d. Shoulder

156. A client has crushing chest pain and ST elevation in leads I, V5, and V6. Which of the following kinds of infarction is the client likely having?
  a. Lateral wall
  b. Inferior wall
  c. Anterior wall
  d. Posterior wall

157. A client is brought to the ED with a hemothorax. A chest tube is to be placed to evacuate the fluid. Which of the following is the proper placement site for a chest tube?
  a. Anterior chest over a rib
  b. Posterior chest under a rib
  c. Lateral chest over a rib
  d. Lateral chest under a rib

158. A 20-year-old client in the ED is seen for a dental abscess. She has markedly severe dental caries and loss of most of her teeth. Use of which drug should be suspected?
  a. LSD
  b. Methamphetamine
  c. Marijuana
  d. Ketamine

159. A client is seen in the ED after an accidental gunshot wound to the jaw. Which of the following is the first priority in treatment?
  a. IV insertion
  b. Airway establishment
  c. Fluid bolus
  d. Exploration for bullet fragments

160. A client is seen with unilateral paralysis of the face with drooling on the side of the mouth and is diagnosed with Bell's palsy. Which cranial nerve is affected in this condition?
  a. I
  b. II
  c. V
  d. VII

161. A client with a history of insulin dependent diabetes is seen with diabetic ketoacidosis (DKA). Which of the following is NOT a common cause of DKA in diabetics?
a. Infection
b. Gastroenteritis
c. Influenza
d. Non-compliance with insulin regimen

162. A 30-year-old client with a fever, heart murmur, and chills is diagnosed with bacterial endocarditis. The patient admits to be a long time IV drug user. Which valve is likely affected?
a. Aortic
b. Pulmonic
c. Tricuspid
d. Mitral

163. A client is seen with an acute migraine headache. The administration of sumatriptan (Imitrex) may be useful. What of the following is NOT a relative contraindication to the administration of Imitrex?
a. Pregnancy
b. Diabetes
c. Uncontrolled hypertension
d. Ischemic heart disease

164. A 3-year-old female forcefully jerked her arm out of her mother's grasp while crossing the street. Since then she is unwilling to move the arm. Which of the following is the most likely pediatric orthopedic disorder?
a. Greenstick fracture
b. Radial head dislocation
c. Wrist dislocation
d. Colles' fracture

165. Following a crush injury, a client has a swollen arm. The surgeon on call has instructed you to report any changes that would indicated that the client needs a fasciotomy. Which of the following is not part of frequent assessments performed for this?
a. Pain
b. Pallor
c. Parasthesia
d. PMI

166. An HIV-infected client who has been not taking his medications presents to the ED with a fever, dry cough, weight loss and diffuse infiltrates on chest xray. What is his most likely diagnosis?
a. Pneumocystis jiroveci pneumonia
b. Hepatitis C
c. Influenza virus infection
d. Parainfluenza virus infection

167. Following a fall from a ladder, a 40-year-old client who sustained a neck injury complains of decreased sensation in his whole body. His HR is 55 and BP is 80/30. He has decreased rectal sphincter tone. Which kind of shock is this client experiencing?
   a. Distributive
   b. Hemorrhagic
   c. Cardiogenic
   d. Respiratory

168. After handling commercial insecticides with his bare hands, a farm worker presents with vomiting, bradycardia, and muscle fasciculations. Which of the following medications can be given to reverse the life-threatening effects of this poison?
   a. Deferoxamine (Desferal)
   b. Atropine
   c. Flumazenil (Romazicon)
   d. Aspirin

169. Which of the following foreign bodies would NOT be visible on an x-ray of a client's arm?
   a. Wood splinter
   b. Plastic splinter
   c. Metal bullet
   d. Shotgun pellet

170. Hair follicles often need to be shaved to allow for close suturing of a laceration. However, which of the following body parts should never be shaved?
   a. Scalp
   b. Eyebrows
   c. Arm
   d. Pubis

171. Which of the following cases would not be at high risk for abnormal wound healing?
   a. 65-year-old diabetic with a scalp laceration
   b. 18-year-old on chronic steroid for sarcoid with an arm laceration
   c. 40-year-old with hypertension and an ankle laceration
   d. 50-year-old morbidly obese female with a scalp laceration

172. A 25-year-old client presents with redness and fluctuance along the side of fingernail and is diagnosed with having a paronychia. Which of the following is the most appropriate treatment for this condition?
   a. Topical antibiotics
   b. Incision and drainage
   c. Warm water soaks
   d. Topical steroid cream

173. A 12-year-old client is seen for a dog bite on the right forearm. He has no medication allergies, and it is determined that antibiotic prophylaxis is needed. Which of the following is the most appropriate antibiotic therapy for this client?

    a. Amoxicillin/clavulanic acid (Augmentin)
    b. Nitrofurantoin (Macrobid)
    c. Fosfomycin (Monurol)
    d. Gentamicin (Garamycin)

174. A thirty-year-old client who went on a missionary trip to Africa two months previously presents to the ED with a history of intermittent fevers. He states that he gets a very high fever up to 104° F that lasts for about 12 hours and then resolves. This occurs about every 3 days. He did not take any medications prior to his trip, as it was "last minute." His initial lab results prompted the lab to call the ED and inform them that he is very anemic. Which of the following is his likely diagnosis?

    a. Liver flukes
    b. Babesiosis
    c. Malaria
    d. Hepatitis

175. A client presents to the ED with a domesticated cat bite. He is worried about contracting rabies. Which of the following animals is the most common animal reservoir for rabies in the United States?

    a. Bats
    b. Hamsters
    c. Mice
    d. Owls

Answer Key and Explanations

1. D: CT provides the best diagnostic method to assess for bleeding if the patient is stable enough to permit. Ultrasound and MRI are not as good methods of imaging in this instance. CBC will not diagnose the source of bleeding.

2. C: Pyloric stenosis, resulting from a stenosis at the pyloric junction, is seen more often in males than females and presents at the six-week time period. Diagnosis is confirmed with ultrasound.

3. B: Blockage of the sphincter of Oddi leads to irritation of the pancreas, leading to pancreatitis.

4. B: Pain in the RLQ with palpation in the LLQ is known as Rovsing's sign and is a diagnostic physical exam sign of appendicitis.

5. D: A nasogastric tube will suction off the acidic contents of the stomach and, if not compensated for, may lead to a metabolic alkalosis.

6. A: A large bore peripheral IV will allow faster fluid delivery than a central line.

7. B: Long-term recent antibiotic use is a common cause for Clostridium difficile due to disruption of the normal colonic flora and overgrowth of this bacterium.

8. B: A bowel perforation will lead to the leakage of air, and this can lead to the visualization of air under the diaphragm on KUB or chest x-ray.

9. C: Elevated WBC is not part of Charcot's triad, which comprises fever, jaundice, and RUQ tenderness. The additional signs of shock and altered mental status make up Reynold's pentad.

10. A: Chronic alcohol abuse can lead to esophageal varices, which can cause profuse upper GI bleeding.

11. C: Crohn's disease is an inflammatory disease that can involve any part of the digestive tract from the mouth to anus, including the stomach.

12. D: The most common cause of LLQ pain in an elderly client is diverticulitis. Appendicitis pain is seen in the RLQ, and Meckel's diverticulum and Hirschsprung's megacolon are both congenital disorders, rarely seen in later adulthood.

13. A: Pain in the RUQ on expiration with palpation is known as Murphy's sign and is suggestive of gallbladder irritation.

14. C: The major goal with all types of heart failure is to prevent further damage and remodeling, prevent exacerbations, and improve the patient's long term prognosis.

15. C: Morphine dilates the venous system, decreasing preload and can improve cardiac output.

16. D: Cardiac tamponade results from the constriction of the heart due to fluid buildup in the pericardial sac, impeding function. Distant heart sounds, distended neck veins, and hypotension are the three components of Beck's triad, a classic sign of cardiac tamponade.

17. A, C, and D: The decision to use PTCA, stents, or CABG is based on multiple factors, including symptoms, severity of CAD, EF, comorbidities, number of blocked arteries, and degree of narrowing of arteries.

18. A: The deciding factor for administration of thrombolytic therapy is the changes in ST elevation in the EKG. As the EKG is a critical determinant for future treatment, it is a primary need early in the care of the patient in the ED.

19. B: This patient needs rate control, so diltizem is indicated, and the patient's blood pressure will be able to support it. The patient has been complaining of these symptoms for longer than 7 days and the patient has not been monitored so ibutilide for cardioversion is not indicated, especially since overall the patient is hemodynamically stable. This patient will need to see a cardiologist for decisions regarding warfarin, cardioversion, or other repairs. Digoxin is only indicated in patients with heart failure.

20. C: Aspirin therapy is not an absolute contraindication to thrombolytic treatment. Active GI bleed, recent hip replacement, and recent hemorrhagic stroke are contraindications.

21. B: As the aorta is not fixed in the body below the aortic arch, a sudden deceleration injury or chest contusion can cause an aortic dissection. The preliminary finding is widening on chest x-ray and a definitive diagnosis is made with an aortogram or CT scan.

22. A: Cardioversion is the treatment of choice for hemodynamically unstable tachycardias.

23. D: Defibrillation is the primary treatment for ventricular fibrillation. As it is the treatment most likely to reverse the condition, it should be used first.

24. C: Atropine is the first line treatment for asystole. If atropine is ineffective, the next drug of choice is epinephrine.

25. A: For inflation of a lung due to pneumothorax, a chest tube is the proper treatment.

26. B: NSAIDs should be avoided in the patient with heart failure especially a patient that is receiving diuretics, as is indicated for heart failure exacerbation, like this patient presents with. NSAIDS impair the body's reaction to diuretics.

27. C: Infectious endocarditis is commonly seen with IV drug users. The use of needles without sterile technique causes seeding of skin bacteria into the bloodstream, and this can then infect the cardiac valves.

28. B: Bedside use of a CO_2 monitor can be used in addition to lung auscultation to assure correct tube placement.

29. C: Ventilation should be stopped briefly before the opening of the pleura so that the lung is not in contact with the chest wall. All the other statements are true about an emergency thoracotomy.

30. B: Sick sinus syndrome is seen in elderly patients, commonly in diabetics, and results from malfunctioning of the AV node.

31. C: 13. The Glasgow Coma Scale is a useful and rapid method of determining level of consciousness in comatose patients, regardless of the cause. The scale is divided into 3 major subgroups: eye opening, best motor response, and best verbal response with point scores for individual responses.

Eye opening	4: Spontaneous. 3: To verbal stimuli. 2: To pain (not of face). 1: No response.
Verbal	5: Oriented. 4: Conversation confused, but can answer questions. 3: Uses inappropriate words. 2: Speech incomprehensible. 1: No response.
Motor	6: Moves on command. 5: Moves purposefully respond pain. 4: Withdraws in response to pain. 3: Decorticate posturing (flexion) in response to pain. 2: Decerebrate posturing (extension) in response to pain. 1: No response.

Injuries/conditions are classified according to the total score: 3-8 Coma; ≤ 8 Severe head injury; 9-12 Moderate head injury; 13-15 Mild head injury.

32. D: A rectal temperature of 100.4° F is considered febrile in pediatric patients.

33. B: Male sex, not female sex is considered a major risk factor for coronary artery disease. Smoking, hypertension, and diabetes are also risk factors.

34. C: This is the classic presentation for epiglottitis. Radiologic confirmation can be made with a lateral x-ray showing swelling in the area. Management of the airway is a priority.

35. B: Benzodiazepines are the most commonly used medications to stop prolonged seizure activity. Lorazepam is one of the commonly given medications to stop status epilepticus because it has a very rapid onset of action. The other two have slower onsets so they would not be beneficial in an emergent situation. Ativan is given every five minutes until the seizures stop or at least until the patient's airway is secured. Sometimes it is given with phenobarbital, but this combination can cause apnea so caution should be used.

36. C: A new onset seizure in an adult of Central or South American descent is likely due to infection with cysticercosis. A pork tapeworm can burrow through the GI tract after ingestion and travel to the brain and cause cysts that can lead to seizure activity.

37. D: After securing the airway, epinephrine can be given subcutaneously to treat anaphylactic shock before an IV has been established. Both diphenhydramine (Benadryl) and corticosteroids can be given IM and IV but not SQ.

38. A: EpiPens are most beneficial when used as soon as the patient has the first symptom. All the other statements are correct ways to use an EpiPen.

39. D: A positive crossed straight leg test is very specific for a herniated disc. To perform the test, the client's leg is extended. A positive finding occurs if the client feels radicular pain in the other leg.

40. A: This is the classic presentation for acute glaucoma. Prompt reduction in the intraocular pressure is needed to preserve vision.

41. D: Thrombolytics are contraindicated in cardiogenic shock that is not secondary to an MI. All other interventions would be appropriate.

42. B: Nuchal rigidity is the chief complain in meningitis and is present in about 75% of this patient population. Lumbar puncture is necessary to obtain cerebral spinal fluid for both diagnostic testing and cultures to determine if the patient has meningitis.

43. A: Daily peak flow measurements should be done by all clients with persistent asthma. Any variation from baseline can provide an early indication of an exacerbation.

44. B: Singulair is used for chronic treatment of asthma but is not a medication for treatment of acute exacerbations. Solu-Medrol, albuterol, and Atrovent are all used in the acute treatment of clients with asthma.

45. A: Theophylline can be used for the treatment of COPD and asthma. It requires regular monitoring for therapeutic levels. Caffiene can exacerbate side effects of the medication. While not absolutely restricted in pregnancy, physicians will need to weight risks and benefits. Moving an appointment back one day would not be a problem, because the patient still got the blood work done and is therefore compliant. Patients using maintenance asthma medications also need to have a rescue inhaler for emergencies.

46. C: Digoxin is used to improve contractility of the myocardium in congestive heart failure. Therapeutic levels are .8 to 2 ng/mL. Therefore these symptoms are not caused by dig toxicity.

47. C: With trauma to the chest and absent or decreased breath sounds, tension pneumothorax is likely. Inflation of the lung can be done with chest tube insertion or with a large needle.

48. A: Women who are pregnant and develop pyelonephritis usually require hospitalization for treatment.

49. C: OTC stimulant laxatives should be avoided if possible because they can lead to dependence and continued problems with constipation in the elderly. Increased exercise, fiber intake, and water intake are all first line treatments for constipation.

50. B: Adenosine usually causes a brief episode of asystole and can be uncomfortable for the patient.

51. D: The presence of thrombocytopenia and ARF makes this multi organ dysfunction syndrome.

52. D: Incidental contact with the brother who has had prior immunization would be permissible for a child with chicken pox. The other family members all have either immunosuppression or pregnancy, which are contraindications for contact with someone with active varicella.

53. C: A current vaccine against Hepatitis C does not exist. Hepatitis A, hepatitis B, and influenza are recommended vaccines for healthcare workers.

54. B: A score of less that 17 on the Mini-Mental Status Exam would indicate severe dementia.

55. D: The sensory part of the trigeminal nerve (cranial nerve V) supplies the anterior two-thirds of the tongue, mouth and jaw area.

56. B: Compromise to the lateral rectus muscle will lead to unopposed action of the antagonizing muscle (medial rectus) and medial deviation with the inability to laterally move the eye.

57. A: Damage to the lower brachial plexus can lead to Erb's palsy with a limp arm and a flexed hand with the palm facing backwards.

58. D: OTC cranberry extract pills can be of benefit in UTI as they acidify the urine and possibly prevent bacterial adhesion to the bladder wall. Extra fluids and frequent voiding is advised. Carbonated sodas will alkalinize the urine, and this can impede improvement.

59. A: A child with a femoral head fracture will likely need surgical fixation to prevent future disability. The other fractures can all be treated with splinting/casting.

60. C: Pulmonary edema (crackles on auscultation) and pedal edema are the most diagnostic physical findings for fluid overload.

61. D: With a high respiratory rate, the patient will blow off excess carbon dioxide (an acid) and, therefore, be at risk for respiratory alkalosis.

62. D: Immediately after any intubation, a chest x-ray is needed to confirm correct placement of the ET tube.

63. C: Often the primary problem with head trauma is a significant increase in swelling, which also interferes with perfusion, causing hypoxia and hypercapnia, which trigger increased blood flow. This increased volume at a time when injury impairs autoregulation increases cerebral edema, which, in turn, increases intracranial pressure and results in a further decrease in perfusion with resultant ischemia. If pressure continues to rise, the brain may herniate.

64. A: Mucomyst is given orally (PO), usually via an NG tube.

65. D: In penetrating trauma to the limb, if arterial damage is possible, the best diagnostic test is an arteriogram.

66. C: An ultrasound is the diagnostic test of choice in testicular torsion, both to evaluate blood flow and evaluate for other causes of the symptoms.

67. D: A Kleihauer-Betke test is a blood test done on the mother to assess for any transmission of fetal blood into the maternal blood stream. It is important to assess for blood type incompatibility issues.

68. B: Spinal headaches from the leak of CSF with lumbar punctures for epidurals can occur. If continuing, a plug can be made from the patient's blood to stop the process.

69. D: MRI tests can cause movement of prior metal implants or clips from prior surgery, so a thorough history about prior surgeries should be done. An MRI of the cervical region will likely not necessitate any contrast dye or shaving.

70. B: The antecubital fossa is the preferred site for obtaining blood for blood cultures.

71. C: An arm or figure-of-eight sling is the most appropriate treatment for uncomplicated clavicle fractures.

72. D: Every ED should have a protocol in place to test the employee for bloodborne pathogens. Notifying the supervisor will allow the protocol to proceed with minimal delay.

73. A: Herpes prophylaxis is not a standard of care after sexual assault. Prophylaxis against HIV, gonorrhea, Chlamydia, and pregnancy are all offered post-sexual assault.

74. C: Medications for erectile dysfunction can cause an unsafe drop in blood pressure when used in conjunction with nitrates.

75. A: The ED supervisor should be notified of such a glaring HIPAA violation as the actions of the MA have placed the hospital in legal jeopardy.

76. C: The injury described is flail chest and it occurs when at least 3 adjacent ribs are fractured, both anteriorly and posteriorly, so that they float free of the rib cage. Treatment includes analgesia, initial stabilization with tape, one side only, don't wrap the chest, and surgical fixation if needed for underlying injury.

77. C: After administration of the Mantoux (PPD) skin test, the skin site should be read within 48 to 72 hours.

78. A: A thoracentesis is done by needle aspiration on the posterior chest wall to both alleviate symptoms and remove fluid for diagnostic testing.

79. D: Tegaderm dressing supply the proper environment for the healing of skin tears, commonly seen in elderly clients.

80. A: Potatoes do not provide a significant source of iron. Animal proteins and spinach are good sources.

81. A: Any client coughing soot and with a hoarse voice should be closely monitored as the person may have respiratory compromise due to damage to the upper respiratory system.

82. B: Smoking, oral contraceptives, and immobilization are all high risk factors that increase the chance of DVT.

83. A: The most common symptom of psychosis is auditory hallucination, usually from an authoritative figure.

84. B: Spiral fractures are the result of extensive twisting force to the bone, and in young children, spiral fractures are usually the result of abuse.

85. D: The rapid shifting of topics with no apparent connections is known as flight of ideas and is a common component of manic states.

86. C: Respiratory disorders cause dyspnea, which can lead to severe anxiety.

87. C: A benzodiazepine, like Ativan, will have an immediate impact on anxiety symptoms. Bupropion, paroxetine, and fluoxetine can take up to 4 to 6 weeks to take effect.

88. C: For issues of placement and discharge, a social worker will have the experience and background to help with planning.

89. B: Potassium must be added to the replacement fluids in clients treated for DKA. During the process, insulin moves glucose into the cells along with potassium, and, if replacement is not done, hypokalemia could result.

90. A: Creatinine is a direct measurement of kidney function and elevation may indicate renal abnormalities. The more muscle mass that you have, the more creatinine you would need to clear, making a higher level possibly acceptable in a young athlete.

91. B: An Allen test is done to assess collateral blood circulation in the hand before performing an ABG on the radial artery.

92. D: Presentation of symptoms hours after a closed head trauma is classic for subdural hematoma. Epidural hematomas usually present with symptoms much sooner due to more rapid bleeding.

93. B: The motor cortex for the right side of the body and speech center is located on the left side of the cerebrum.

94. A: Adult males have the highest success rates among those who attempt suicide. This is likely due to the higher use of firearms with males, compared to other less-effective methods.

95. D: Tricyclic medications, such as Elavil, can cause QT prolongation and cardiac abnormalities.

96. D: Norepinephrine is the antibiotic of choice in septic shock.

97. D: Nifedipine (Procardia) has been found to increase the risk of stroke due to rapid hypotension and is not recommended for treatment of hypertensive urgencies.

98. B: Asplenic clients (either from splenectomy or auto-infarction from sickle cell disease) should be vaccinated with the pneumococcal vaccine.

99. B: Clients with infectious mononucleosis can develop splenomegaly and should avoid contact sports until cleared by their primary care provider.

100. C: Proteinuria and hypertension are the hallmarks of pre-eclampsia, and all pregnant clients in the ED should have a urinalysis done if presenting with a headache.

101. C: An INR level of 2.5 to 3.5 indicates an appropriate level of anticoagulation for a mechanical heart valve.

102. B: The mean corpuscular volume (MCV) measures the size of the red blood cells and is an indicator of the kind of anemia present.

103. D: An interosseous line, a large bore needle into the anterior tibia, can provide rapid infusion of fluids in a trauma situation in young children. Central lines are not ideal in rapid fluid infusion due to the length of the line and size of the cannula.

104. B: Kayexalate is a resin that binds to potassium in the GI tract and can decrease potassium levels until dialysis can be arranged.

105. A: Azithromycin has good antibiotic coverage against streptococcal organisms. Nafcillin and Amoxil are both penicillin derivatives and should be avoided. Ciprofloxacin does not have optimal coverage for this infection.

106. D: Because LBBB obscures the EKG findings in the lateral leads, so this can make the determination whether to give thrombolytics difficult. The determination to give thrombolytics is based on ST elevation in the lateral leads.

107. B: Long-term use of older anti-psychotic medications like haloperidol (Haldol) can lead to the development of tardive dyskinesia.

108. C: Spinal cord injury without radiographic abnormality (SCIWORA) occurs when, due to flexibility of the cervical spine in children, they have a neurological injury without radiographic evidence.

109. D: Flumazenil (Romazicon) is an antagonist medication that can be used to reverse the effects of benzodiazepine overdose.

110. B: Ethanol can be used as a competitive inhibitor to prevent the toxic metabolites of ethylene glycol ingestion.

111. C: Fresh frozen plasma (FFP) can be given to rapidly reverse the consequences of over anti-coagulation.

112. A: Cocaine use can cause coronary events even in very young clients.

113. C: This is known as Finkelstein's test and is diagnostic for tendonitis at the base of the thumb.

114. B: Trichotillomania is the psychiatric condition in which a client intentionally pulls out his/her own hair, usually seen in adolescent females.

115. A: Marfan's syndrome is an inherited connective tissue disease that can lead to tall stature, increased risk for aortic aneurysms, and retinal problems.

116. B: The visual cortex is located in the posterior cerebrum, and damage to this area can lead to vision deficits.

117. B: In the ABC acronym, if airway has been cared for breathing should be assessed and addressed next. This patient is at risk for breathing difficulties due to risk for aspiration pneumonia, and unknown time down.

118. B: A Thompson test is used to assess for structural integrity of the calf muscle.

119. D: Tetanus boosters are recommended every 10 years for adults.

120. B: Defibrillation is the curative treatment for ventricular fibrillation and should be administered as soon as possible. The shock can be administered at any time during the cardiac cycle. Because the prompt specifies that this is a biphasic defibrillator, you know that the shock will be between 100-200 J. Monophasic defibrillators (much less common in practice today), deliver a shock between 200-360 J.

121. B: A 1% burn to the dorsal thigh can usually be treated medically. Burns to the hand, face, and genitals can all cause significant impairment; so even with only a 1% body surface area, prompt consultation with a plastic surgeon is indicated.

122. A: The client with an open chest wound likely has a pneumothorax, a quickly treatable condition that if ignored can lead to respiratory collapse, and should be treated first. The client with the open head wound and no pulse is likely beyond saving and potentially savable clients should be seen first.

123. C: An intravenous pyelogram (IVP) is the gold standard test of choice in testing for kidney stones.

124. B: Vitamin K is used to reverse the effects of Coumadin but has no place in the treatment of a sickle cell crisis. Oxygen, IV hydration, and pain medication are all first line therapies for a sickle cell crisis.

125. B: These are all classic symptoms of superior vena cava syndrome in which a tumor or mass is impeding the venous return to the heart.

126. A: Hyperkalemia is noted to cause tall, peaked T-waves on EKG. The physician would likely order a beside potassium and then treat with calcium gluconate IV to decrease the cardiac effects.

127. D: Overproduction of thyroid hormone can lead to tachycardia, weight loss, and fatigue.

128. C: Orbital cellulitis needs to be aggressively treated as the venous drainage system for the orbits is through the cavernous sinus of the brain and can lead to meningitis if not treated promptly.

129. C: These are symptoms of leukemia. Further workup will be needed.

130. D: The patient has salicylate poisoning, found in aspirin and pepto bismol. Acetylcysteine is for Tylenol poisoning and 4 tylenol pm would not call for this treatment. The other treatments listed are indicated in salicylate poisoning.

131. C: The most important ED action for patients with food poisoning or other GI illnesses is an evaluation for degree of dehydration to determine if oral or IV courses of fluids are necessary.

132. A: If a client has never been given the tetanus vaccine, coverage for a wound can be supplied with the tetanus immunoglobulin until immunity is achieved from the vaccine.

133. D: Gardasil vaccine protects against the human papilloma virus (HPV), which can lead to genital warts, cervical dysplasia, and cervical cancer.

134. C: The incidence of concomitant infection with chlamydia can be as high as 50% in those infected with gonorrhea, so clients should always be treated for both organisms.

135. B: This bull's-eye rash is a classic presentation for Lyme disease, which should be treated with antibiotics to avoid systemic complications.

136. A: A herpes zoster rash on the face extending to the tip of the nose may involve the ophthalmic branch of the facial nerve and can lead to possible eye complication, including blindness. Prompt consultation with an ophthalmologist is prudent.

137. B: Cardiac arrhythmias are the most common cause of death after electrical injuries. Clients should have a thorough cardiac examination, including EKG and enzyme tests.

138. B: Q-T interval prolongation and J-waves (Osborn waves) occur in hypothermic conditions as clients become poikilothermic and cannot rewarm themselves.

139. D: Acetazolamide can be used to both to prevent and alleviate the symptoms of acute mountain sickness (AMS). Dexamethasone has also been used in the treatment of this condition.

140. A: Parainfluenza viruses are the causative organisms in most cases of croup. The treatment is supportive, based on symptoms, and antibiotics are not usually indicated.

141. C: Meckel's diverticulum is caused by the abnormal collection of gastric cells in the lower intestine and is the most common cause of painless lower GI bleeding in a child.

142. A: Erythema infectiosum (Fifth disease) is caused by parvovirus B19 and is characterized by a fever and "slapped cheek" rash.

143. B: The symptoms described, especially enlarged spleen would likely lead the physician to order an antibody test like the Monospot test to detect antibodies in the course of infectious mononucleosis. It is most accurate in the third week of disease.

144. D: Coronary artery disease due to arteritis or aneurysm is the most significant complication of Kawasaki's disease. A cardiac evaluation is absolutely necessary.

145. B: Aspirin use in children during febrile illnesses has been linked to the development of Reye syndrome, so its use is discouraged in these circumstances.

146. A: Venous cutdowns are done at the ankle area to visually insert a cannula into a vein and start IV fluids.

147. B: Le Fort fractures are mid-face fractures involving the maxilla to some extent and are graded I, II, or III, depending on the bones involved. All of the interventions could be appropriate at some point in this patient's care, but the most important one is assisting the physician to safely assess the patient. Suctioning may be needed to keep the airway patent due to bleeding. Otoscopes and other equipment will likely be needed. This assessment will guide further decisions and treatment.

148. B: Impingement or irritation to the median nerve leads to symptoms on the volar radial side of the hand, known as carpal tunnel syndrome.

149. A: Tenderness in the anatomical snuffbox of the wrist is suggestive of a scaphoid fracture, the most commonly fractured carpal bone.

150. D: Ectopic pregnancy is a potentially life-threatening condition that should be considered in all women of childbearing age. A beta-HCG blood test for pregnancy is standard in the abdominal lab workup for females.

151. C: A barium enema would not only be diagnostic of intussusception but also potentially curative in reducing the involution of the bowel.

152. D: Parainfluenza virus mainly affects the upper respiratory tract and is not implicated in pancreatitis. Alcohol abuse, gallstones, and hypertriglyceridemia are all common causes of pancreatitis.

153. A: Benzodiazepines, such as Ativan, are the mainstay of treatment for alcohol withdrawal and the prevention of withdrawal seizures.

154. B: Diaphragmatic irritation that causes left shoulder pain is known as Kehr's sign and is usually caused by splenic bleeding.

155. B: Lumbar spinal compression fractures are common from compression type injuries to the lower legs and should be evaluated closely.

156. A: A lateral wall infarction would lead to ST elevation in I, V5 and V6.

157. C: A chest tube is placed in the lateral chest over a rib. As the neurovascular bundle runs inferiorly to each rib, care is taken to slip over the top of each rib to prevent nerve damage.

158. B: The use of methamphetamine is often associated with "meth mouth," a marked deterioration in dental health due to the drug. Methamphetamine use can lead to decreased saliva and grinding of the teeth (bruxism), causing this condition.

159. B: With any trauma patient, airway is the first priority and should be addressed before any other intervention.

160. D: The VII (seventh) cranial nerve is affected in Bell's palsy, a post-viral condition that is usually transient.

161. C: Influenza usually does not cause DKA. Any condition that increases blood sugar levels (non-compliance, infection) or decreases fluid and food intake (gastroenteritis) can commonly lead to DKA in diabetics.

162. C: The use of contaminated needles can seed the bloodstream with bacteria and lead to bacterial endocarditis. The right side of the heart is usually most affected, as this is where the blood goes to first, with the tricuspid valve being the most commonly effected.

163. B: Triptan medications, such as Imitrex may be used with diabetes. Pregnancy, uncontrolled hypertension and ischemic heart disease are all relative contraindications to the use of triptan medications.

164. B: A twisting type injury is the common cause for a radial head dislocation (nursemaid's elbow). Gentle supination while flexing the elbow with pressure on the radial head will usually reduce the dislocation and produce a palpable "clunk" for the examiner.

165. D: A crush injury can lead to swelling of the tissues causing a compartment syndrome, leading to decreased blood flow to the distal extremity. In assessing neurostatus of an extremity, use the 5 Ps- pain, pallor, paresthesia, paralysis, and pulse.

166. A: This is the classic presentation for Pneumocystis jirovecii pneumonia. Since the advent of anti-retroviral therapy, incidence has decreased.

167. A: A history of trauma with a HR not compensating for a low BP is indicative of neurogenic shock, a type of distributive shock.

168. B:Atropine can be given to reverse the potentially life-threatening bradycardia that can result from organophosphate poisoning.

169. A: Wood or other plant-based foreign bodies are not routinely visible on plain x-ray. They are visible on mammogram, and this modality can be used in difficult cases.

170. B: Eyebrows should never be shaved as they often do not grow back, and their edges are used to approximate the wound.

171. C: Hypertension does not increase the risk of abnormal wound healing. Diabetes, steroid use, and morbid obesity are all risk factors for poor wound healing.

172. B: Incision and drainage (I&D) is the most appropriate treatment for paronychia and is usually the only therapy needed.

173. A: Augmentin is the drug of choice in animal bites. The antibiotic chosen must provide good coverage of Gram-negative and anaerobic organisms.

174. C: Relapsing, intermittent high fevers with anemia and intracellular parasites seen on peripheral blood smear are highly suggestive of malaria. Babesiosis is also an intracellular parasite causing anemia and fever but is mainly found in New England.

175. A: Bats are the most common reservoir for rabies in the United States. Other wild mammals, such as raccoons and skunks, can also carry the virus. It is very uncommon in rodents.